Letters of Appreciation from U.S. Government Leaders

"I want to take this opportunity to thank [Earl Updike] for [his] book . . . I look forward to working with [Earl Updike] for a better future for our country."

Al Gore
Vice President of the United States, Washington, DC

"I was happy to see that the Department of Agriculture recently revised the Food Guide Pyramid to encourage plant food consumption. I agree with [Earl Updike] that eating healthy foods is a critical part of health care reform. I think more and more people are beginning to recognize this.

Patricia Schroeder
U.S. Congresswoman, Washington, DC

". . . Our present system of health care delivery is extremely complicated. We currently spend over $800 billion per year on medical care—over 13 percent of our Gross National Product. . . . changes are needed. [Earl Updike's] comments on the importance of prevention are right on target. Much study has proven that preventative health efforts produce both a healthier population and reduce health care expenditures. Making intelligent lifestyle choices is one of the most important factors in this effort, and it is clear that the value of a healthy diet is extremely high."

Dan Schaefer
Member of U.S. Congress, Washington, DC

"I couldn't agree more with [Earl Updike] about the importance of preventative health care and healthful living and eating habits as major contributors to holding down health care costs."

Jim Kolbe
Member of U.S. Congress

"My wife and I have enjoyed [Earl Updike's] book. We have already tried two of the recipes. [His] book will give me a guide as to a better diet."

Harry Reïd
United States Senate

"Like [Earl Updike], I believe prevention is key in our attempts to solve the health care crisis in our country. I also believe [Earl] when [he] says that a healthy, fortified diet is the first place to start.

John T. Doolittle
4th District, California, Congress of the United States

"Health care and adequate nutrition for everyone is very much on the minds of all of us these days. [Earl Updike is] making a valiant contribution, and I salute [his] effort."

David E. Skaggs
U.S. House of Representatives, Washington, DC

"This book promises to be insightful, and is timely, since our nation has renewed its concentration on health care. It will be a welcome addition to my library."

Dirk Kempthorne
United States Senate

"By reducing the amount of animal fats and replacing them with fruits, vegetables, and cereals, the result is a diet rich in fiber and protein that reduces the risk of heart disease. Clearly, nutrition education is important for both children and adults to prevent serious health problems and health care costs in the future.

Nancy Landon Kassebaum
United States Senate

"[I thank Earl Updike] for writing and sharing [his] views on health care reform."

Hillary Rodham Clinton
The White House

The Miracle Diet

Easy Permanent Weight Loss

14 days to New Vigor and Health

Fat Free	Cholesterol Free	High Fiber

Oatmeal Soup (mexican)
1 c oatmeal
   chicken stock
   vegies - Any Kind
   garlic
   tomato?
   peppers
   onions
   carrots
   celery
   spices
Basically any flavorful stock w/ veggies
+ oatmeal.

The Miracle Diet
Best Possible Health 1995

For information address:

**Best Possible Health
P.O.Box 54282
Phoenix, AZ 85078-4282
1-800-922-9681**

ISBN 1-887437-00-2 Softback edition

Distributed by
Best Possible Health
P.O.Box 54282
Phoenix, AZ 85078-4282
1-800-922-9681

Cover design by Wil Crandall
Lithographed in the United States of America
Typesetting by Paula Conway

"For the Best Possible Health"

The Miracle Diet

Easy

Permanent Weight Loss

Fat Free	Cholesterol Free	High Fiber

- Eat all you want

- Never be hungry

- Lose up to 10 lbs. per month

- Learn how Fat makes **you** Fat

- Avoid the killers Cholesterol and Fat!

- Become a **Plantarian**

14 days to New Vigor and Health

LOOK BETTER . . . FEEL BETTER
SAVE MONEY ON FOOD
SAVE MONEY ON MEDICAL / DENTAL
LOSE WEIGHT PERMANENTLY
INCREASE YOUR ENERGY

Earl F. Updike

Foreword by **Neal D. Barnard, M.D.**
President, national Physicians Committee For Responsible Medicine
Author of "The Power of Your Plate" and "Food For Life."

"The doctor of the future will give no medicine, but will interest his patient in the care of the human frame, in diet and in the cause and prevention of disease."

—Thomas A. Edison

"Let food be thy medicine."

—Hippocrates ca. 431 B.C.

Dedication

To all those who desire the *"Best Possible Health,"* and especially to the memory of my late wife, Ethel, who was my best friend and love for 49 years. She formulated most of these recipes and made me promise to write this book.

Acknowledgments

I gratefully give thanks to my editor, Jim Catano, who believes in good health for everyone. I appreciate so much my friend and medical advisor, Kenneth E. Johnson Sr., M.D., who guided me all the way. Thanks to my son, Alan, who encouraged me to write this book to share this life-saving information with everyone.

I give special thanks to author, researcher, and world renowned authority on health and nutrition, John McDougall, M.D., who has been my inspiration for more than ten years. Dr. McDougall's four books, audio tapes, video tapes, TV programs, and lectures have had a major impact on the health attitudes of health professionals and laymen in America and throughout the world. Nutritional pioneer, Nathan Pritikin, started a health revolution in the 1970s and now many scientific health experts and writers espouse eating plant foods in place of animal foods.

Thanks to Dr. Neal Barnard and the national Physicians Committee For Responsible Medicine for the **"New Four Food Groups"**. This guide is a major breakthrough for better health for everyone.

Finally, many thanks to Cheri Updike, my new bride and new inspiration. She has spent numerous hours, advising, proofreading, and cheering me on to the completion of this book.

The New Four Food Groups will prove to be the most important scientific medical disclosure for the *"Best Possible Health,"* in the twentieth century.

The New Four Food Groups was announced April 8, 1991, by the Physicians Committee for Responsible Medicine, P.O. Box 6322, Washington, D.C. 20016. (202) 686-2210

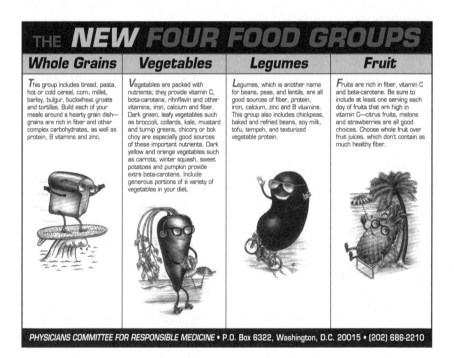

THE NEW FOUR FOOD GROUPS

Whole Grains	Vegetables	Legumes	Fruit
This group includes bread, pasta, hot or cold cereal, corn, millet, barley, bulgur, buckwheat groats and tortillas. Build each of your meals around a hearty grain dish—grains are rich in fiber and other complex carbohydrates, as well as protein, B vitamins and zinc.	Vegetables are packed with nutrients; they provide vitamin C, beta-carotene, riboflavin and other vitamins, iron, calcium and fiber. Dark green, leafy vegetables such as broccoli, collards, kale, mustard and turnip greens, chicory or bok choy are especially good sources of these important nutrients. Dark yellow and orange vegetables such as carrots, winter squash, sweet potatoes and pumpkin provide extra beta-carotene. Include generous portions of a variety of vegetables in your diet.	Legumes, which is another name for beans, peas, and lentils, are all good sources of fiber, protein, iron, calcium, zinc and B vitamins. This group also includes chickpeas, baked and refried beans, soy milk, tofu, tempeh, and texturized vegetable protein.	Fruits are rich in fiber, vitamin C and beta-carotene. Be sure to include at least one serving each day of fruits that are high in vitamin C—citrus fruits, melons and strawberries are all good choices. Choose whole fruit over fruit juices, which don't contain as much healthy fiber.

PHYSICIANS COMMITTEE FOR RESPONSIBLE MEDICINE • P.O. Box 6322, Washington, D.C. 20015 • (202) 686-2210

Vitamin B12

If you are pregnant or nursing, or if you follow this program strictly for more than three years, then take at least 5 micrograms supplemental Vitamin B12 each day.

CAUTION

The information in this book is meant to educate you regarding better health and happiness. Any decision you make in the treatment of any illness should include the advice of a physician experienced in the effects of dietary change. If you are seriously ill or on medication, do not change your diet without your doctor's or health professional's approval .

Definition of "FAT FREE"

The food industry has generally adopted the phrase "Fat Free" to mean no added fat. There is naturally occurring fat in low-fat plant foods such as: beans (3%), rice (4%), corn (8%), whole wheat flour (5%), potatoes (trace).

There is no added fat in any recipe in this book. All plant foods contain some fat even if it is only a trace. There are only five plant foods that contain high fat. They are: avocados, nuts, olives, coconut and milk chocolate, none of which are used in these recipes. Some soy products are high in fat.

RECIPE STATISTICS

We do not spell out fat grams, cholesterol mg., carbohydrate grams, protein grams or fiber grams because:

- The fat content in these recipes is ideal, averaging between 5 and 10%.
- There is no cholesterol in any recipe.
- Protein averages out at about 10% (ideal).
- Complex carbohydrate averages about 80% (ideal).
- These recipes supply about 40 to 60 grams of fiber a day (ideal).

TABLE OF CONTENTS

FOREWORD

In medical school and in my years of research and practice I have seen overwhelming evidence that foods, when properly chosen, can truly work wonders. In this volume, Earl Updike shows how to put this knowledge to work. He had translated complex and powerful medical principles into easy, practical steps that you can use to slim down, boost your energy, and get healthy, or stay that way.

For many people, that will mean getting back into clothes they hadn't been able to wear in years, or looking great at a high school reunion or holiday get-together, instead of struggling and failing with old-fashioned calorie-counting diets. For others, it will mean impressing their doctors with a stunningly low cholesterol level, a blood pressure that has returned to normal almost like magic, or a reduced need for medication—perhaps no need for it at all. And for many people, it will mean the difference between a life cut short by serious illness and one that is actually expanded and filled with energy.

I have long been enthusiastic about Earl Updike's ability to assemble a wealth of information and delicious, practical recipes into the most user-friendly books available anywhere. This book is his best ever—a book which I would like to see on every kitchen table and in every doctor's office. When that happens, a doctor's job will be much, much easier, and people in all walks of life will have more power to determine their level of health and vitality than they could have ever imagined.

As you read this volume, please share what you learn with others, so that they can take advantage of it, too.

Neal D. Barnard, M.D.
President, Physicians Committee for Responsible Medicine
Washington, D.C.
Author of "The Power of Your Plate" and "Food For Life."

xiii

For the perfect combination
you need our cookbook with nearly
400 Fat Free-Cholesterol Free-
High Fiber Recipes.
Look for the bright red cover!

"THE MIRACLE DIET COOKBOOK"

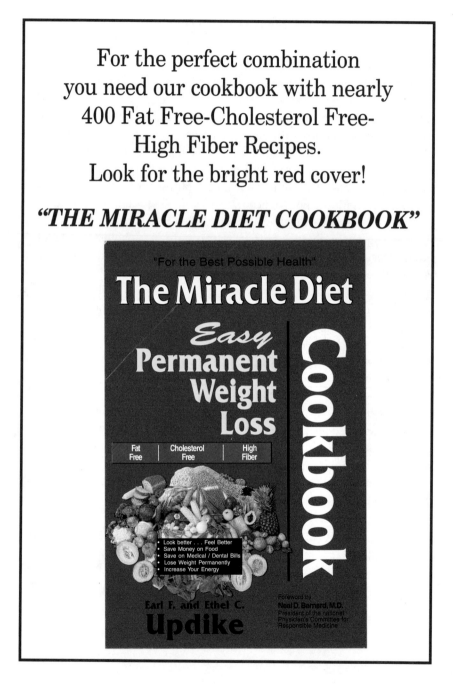

INTRODUCTION

At age five, I announced to my parents that I wanted to be a medical doctor so I could help sick people and find the cause of disease. Although my interest in medicine continued as I grew, I eventually followed my father's business instead. However, I never lost the desire to discover what causes people to suffer from heart disease, cancer, diabetes, stroke, and other degenerative diseases. By 1962, age forty, I had decided diet must have a great effect on the cause of the major diseases and I began reading everything I could find about health and nutrition.

In 1973, Dr. Denis Burkitt, a world-renowned medical researcher and scientist, proclaimed that Americans and other Westerners needed to drastically increase dietary fiber many times.[1] Dr. Burkitt said recently "Our ancestors ate over 100 grams of fiber per day. Each person ate 1 1/4 pounds of whole grain bread per day, but today each person eats less than 1/4 pound of (mostly white) bread, per day." He said we need to greatly increase our intake of whole grain bread.[2]

In 1979 Nathan Pritikin, an electronics genius, wrote *The Pritikin Program for Diet and Exercise.* Over two decades earlier doctors had told Pritikin that he had incurable heart disease. He immediately began looking for foods that could prevent, or even cure, heart disease and other conditions. His book revealed that a plant-based diet without any added fat (vegetable or animal) enables the arteries to heal themselves of atherosclerosis.

Since 1979, there has been an avalanche of information confirming the direct relationship between the food we eat and the degenerative diseases from which we suffer and die. These conditions include coronary heart disease, cancer, diabetes, stroke, high blood pressure, kidney disease, and many other modern-day scourges.

Over the past sixteen years, it has become increasingly clear that the consumption of animal products (chicken, fish, red meat, dairy products, and eggs) causes obesity and disease, while the eating of plant foods creates lean bodies, health, strength, and well-being. The 1992 US Department of Agriculture Food Guide Pyramid confirms the need for mostly plant foods in our diet.

Today we are continually reminded to cut down on cholesterol and fats and to boost the amount of fiber in our diet. That's easy when you change to a Plantarian (plant-centered) diet. Plants contain no cholesterol, very little fat, and lots of fiber.

You'll find easy to use "how-to" information in this book. If you apply it, you will lose weight, enjoy better health and quality of life, however it will make your "wallet fatter."

That is only part of what you will find in these pages. You'll also learn the negative impact of animal foods and high fat on your health.

Consider, for example what is happening to our nation's children. Over the past twenty years, the mean weight of American children and adolescents has increased dramatically; in direct proportion to the increase in fat intake and cholesterol levels. These changes are caused by high-fat foods and cholesterol-laden animal products that many parents allow their children to eat early in life. American children are now at much greater risk of developing heart disease, stroke, cancer, diabetes, high blood pressure, and many other degenerative diseases and of doing so earlier in life.[3]

So go ahead. Read the latest scientific information about diet and health. The *"miracle"* of The "Miracle Diet" is the power that it gives you to enjoy "the Best Possible Health." This condition, to which I'll refer regularly, has blessed several entire civilizations throughout history. Modern science is beginning to understand this, and this book gives you the key to enjoy the miracle. The chapters that follow will show you how to be healthier, happier, and more loving than you ever dreamed possible!

—EARL F. UPDIKE

One

Easy, Permanent Weight Loss

Americans Are Getting Fatter! The average American today packs around eight pounds more than he or she did a decade ago.

Seventy-one percent of Americans are overweight, up from fifty-eight percent in 1983 according to a 1995 Harris Poll.

Diets don't work in the long run, as many of you already know. As many as 97% of all people who go on expensive commercial diets regain all of the lost weight and many even put on additional fat. Of course, to the experienced "calorie counter" this information is not news.

The reason dieters are plagued with such poor weight-loss success is that they are eating the wrong fuel (food). Just cutting down on the consumption of high-fat animal foods and added animal and vegetable fats simply does **NOT** work for most people.

Dieting, or cutting your calorie intake, is a self-imposed state of starvation. Eventually, you tire of starving yourself and begin satisfying your natural hunger drive with the same old, high-fat, animal foods.

Consider, too, the powerful advertising industry. The purveyors of popular food items do not want you to know the health consequences of eating their products. We are given only half truths in advertising, in the news, and even as medical advice, and we continue to eat tons of animal foods and other high-fat items.

The industrial giants know that if the whole truth were known, the outcry would shake this nation's food and medical complex.

What's New?

Revolutionary truths have been discovered during the past few decades about food and health. We have made fantastic break-throughs in human nutrition. Scientific literature is now full of ir-refutable evidence that proves plant foods create health, while ani-mal foods and added fat create disease, suffering, and death.

Plant food is generally very low in fat, high in complex carbohy-drates, high in fiber, and contains absolutely no cholesterol. There are only five commonly used, high-fat plant foods: olives (98 percent fat), avocados (88 percent fat), coconuts (92 percent fat), most nuts and seeds (75 to 90 percent fat), and chocolate (milk chocolate is 56 percent fat). Some soy products also are high in fat.

Animal foods, such as chicken, fish, red meat, dairy products and eggs, are all laden with huge amounts of saturated fat and cholesterol. Red meats (beef, pork, mutton), egg yolks and dairy products account for three-fourths of the saturated fats Americans eat. Hamburger is the single major contributor, and cheese holds the number two posi-tion. One cheeseburger can be equivalent to eating 13 pats of butter. This leads to hundreds of thousands of heart-attack deaths each year. And there is absolutely **NO** fiber in any animal product.

So What Is A Truly Balanced Diet?

The **"New Four Food Groups"** (Whole Grains, Legumes, Vegetables and Fruits) announced in April 1991 by the Physicians Committee For Responsible Medicine promotes optimum health. Animal foods and fats, promoted in the old outdated "Basic Four Food Groups" have not only been discredited but have been proven to be harmful.[1]

Scientific literature now indicates that plant foods constitute a *"truly balanced diet."* Contrast that to previous claims by our own government between 1956 and 1992, that *"a balanced diet"* consists of mostly meats, cheeses, eggs, and dairy products—in other words, animal foods, fats, and cholesterol. The animal and dairy industries have promoted that belief for 80 years. Now we know that such "balance" is responsible for a virtual epidemic of coronary heart disease, coronary artery disease, high blood pressure, stroke, diabetes, cancer, and more. In the pages that follow, you'll read the scientific documentation that proves this claim.[2]

But that's not all, you'll also learn how to protect yourself against these diseases. You'll discover how to free your body from cholesterol, excess fat, excessive pesticides, artificial hormones, and the other harmful elements of that so-called "balanced diet."

The book you hold in your hands can change your life **IF** you let it. It can change the lives of your loved ones. As you learn the truth about the food you eat, you'll learn how your diet holds great power and you'll learn how to harness that power.

You may be thinking that old habits are difficult to break and worrying that giving up your old eating habits will make you feel deprived. Don't worry! You'll learn to savor foods that are healthy, easy to prepare, nourishing, and best of all, delicious! You'll discover that the *real* deprivation comes from feeding your body foods that cause disease and death.

It's easy to change your lifestyle when, in your mind's eye, you can perceive the fabulous benefits you'll enjoy. Just imagine a slim, attractive body and no more yo-yo dieting. Your body's immune system will be at its best protecting you from dreaded diseases like heart disease, cancer, diabetes, etc.

"It's all in your mind," psychologists say "you can change any habit in 21 days." Change your fuel—become a "Plantarian" and before 21 days are up your body will thank you for it!

What Is A Plantarian?

The Miracle Diet is a plant-centered diet program that allows your body to seek its ideal weight with natural, high energy. It is based upon plants, not just vegetables, Five basic starches are the basis of the diet.

- **Grain**   (wheat, oats, and barley)
- **Rice**   (another basic grain)
- **Corn**   (another basic grain)
- **Legumes**   (beans, peas, and lentils)
- **Potatoes**   (the only vegetable)

This is a "Plantarian," Not a Vegetarian Program

plan•tar'•i•an (plan tar' ian) n. [plant + arian] a person whose basic diet revolves around plants (starches), supplemented with vegetables and fruit.

Easy permanent weight loss is only one of the fantastic rewards that come to you after you become a "Plantarian." Plant eaters, "Plantarians" are significantly trimmer than meat-eaters.

Commit yourself to try a 14-day experiment. Most people try starvation diets for much longer than two weeks. Changing to the correct fuel (plant food) is so easy and satisfying. Now you can eat as much as you want of the right foods instead of starving yourself. And just imagine, you can lose weight at the same time!

It's so simple. All you have to do is change your thinking about food. Remember: a plant-centered diet is the correct fuel for man and we thrive on it.

Scientific studies have proved that cutting calories works permanently only about 3% of the time. This of course is not news to you! Perhaps you've tried starving yourself by cutting and counting calories and you've already proved to yourself that it just doesn't work in the long run. Perhaps you have tried different commercial diets. You may have lost and regained weight many times. This can be very discouraging. The purpose of this book is to give you new hope and encouragement.

Oprah Winfrey Says

Oprah Winfrey is a great example that supermarket fad diets do not work. She finally learned the secret to success is to *"ZAP THE FAT."* Get it out of your life! How do you do that? Become a "Plantarian!" Eat a plant-centered diet where little fat exists.

Oprah is now teaching millions of viewers her secret for permanent weight loss.

ONE: Eat only 20 grams of fat per day. (Approximately 10% fat calories.)

TWO: Drink at least 8 glasses of water per day.

THREE: Make sure you eat your last meal early enough to digest it fully before turning in for the night.

FOUR: No cocktails. Eliminate alcohol. Drinking is a no-no because it slows down your metabolism.

FIVE: Eat five servings of fruit and vegetables every day.

SIX: Eat three meals and two snacks a day. She says, "Dieting doesn't work." (*Star,* May 16, 1995).

Plants are naturally very low in fat with few exceptions, which you will learn about as you read this book. You will also learn that low-calorie (starvation) diets are not "natural". They add to the dilemma of obesity by actually causing additional weight gain.

It's not "natural" to be overweight. Three billion people on this planet are lean and healthy from living on a plant-centered diet.

When you consume a plant-centered (Plantarian) diet of grains, beans, vegetables and fruits, your fat intake will be 10% or less. For overweight people this is the *"key"* to weight control.

The traditional fatty diets of America and of other affluent countries are not "natural". The typical American gets 40% or more of his or her calories from fat—four times the amount the body needs. This is why people, as a whole, in this country are continuing to gain weight at a rapidly increasing rate.

As stated before, a Harris pole reveals that in 1983, 58% of Americans were overweight whereas now in 1995, 71% of our countrymen are overweight. To make it plainer, the average weight of Americans has risen 8 pounds in little more than a decade.

Being overweight is not just a cosmetic issue, it is clearly linked to cancer, diabetes, heart disease, and many other health problems.

Erroneous Myths about Diets

Why are we gaining all of this weight in spite of over 30 billion dollars being spent annually on fad diets? Because people have the following *erroneous beliefs:*

1. **That we must dramatically cut calories to control weight.**

2. **That if we eat too much, it will make us fat.**

3. **That the problem is merely a lack of "character" or "discipline."**

4. **That we're better off eating chicken, turkey, and fish than red meat.**

5. **That a high protein diet is healthy.**

6. **That vegetable shortening and oil are healthier than animal fat.**

7. **That the greatest danger in eating candy, cookies, rich desserts and junk foods is the sugar content not the fat.**

These erroneous beliefs cause us to fail in our quest for naturally slim, attractive bodies.

Americans are confused as to why obesity is so prevalent. Commercial diet programs that seem to have success initially almost always fail. The reason for our dilemma is that we don't understand how the body controls weight. We do not understand how to control our lifestyle so that we can both lose weight and maintain a new attractive body. If you want to be successful, you are going to have to change a few outdated ideas on eating.

As for the myth that heavy people eat more than thin people, scientists now say it's just the opposite. Thin people eat more calories per pound of body weight than fat people. Calories are a consideration but overall they are not the cause of obesity in our affluent society. For most people, overweight is **not** caused by **how much** we eat but by **what we eat.**

Before anyone can achieve lasting success in controlling weight at healthful levels, he or she must become convinced that *obesity is not caused by eating too much!* If this were true, we would expect that people who consume more calories would be the most overweight. This is not the case according to many scientific studies. The excess calorie theory simply does not hold up under scrutiny.

When societies with little or no obesity (such as China) are compared to those societies with epidemic obesity (such as the U.S.), it is found that people in the "thin" societies consume many more calories per pound of body weight than those in fat societies. The Chinese consume about 2700 calories per person per day compared to 2400 calories per day for Americans. Nevertheless, they are about 25% thinner.

Another myth still believed by many people today is that carbohydrates are fattening. It's not the potatoes, rice, and pasta that's fattening, it's the greasy toppings of butter, sour cream, grated cheese and bacon bits that expand our hips and bellies. Actually carbohydrates are very important for permanent weight control, they contain only 4 calories per gram.

Noted health authority, Dr. Marc Sorenson, says, "Obesity is not caused by overeating, nor is it caused by consuming too many calories. Obesity results from high-fat nutrition, failure to exercise, and intermittent starvation programs commonly called "diets." Research has established conclusively that fat people eat no more than, and in most instances considerably less than, thin people."

"FAT PEOPLE DIET AND BECOME FATTER.
A primary cause of obesity then is UNDEREATING."

Restricted calorie dieting has been and continues to be a futile and debilitating waste of time. Nevertheless, both the diet industry and the American waistline continue to expand.

Dr. Sorenson continues, "Yes, dieting causes obesity. Those who eat less will ultimately have a higher percentage of body fat than those who eat more. Dieting is, in fact, the very best method of causing obesity especially when combined with such other factors as high-fat nutrition and sedentary living."[3]

Guaranteed Failure

Trying to lose weight by dramatically lowering your calorie intake will nearly guarantee failure. You will be frustrated and even heavier in the long run.

Expensive near-starvation programs, costing hundreds of dollars per month, don't work for long-term weight loss or weight control. Even worse, these starvation diets set the stage for more severe weight problems as the years go by.

Why Doesn't Dieting Work?

Low calorie dieting disrupts the body's metabolism. When you deprive yourself of food as you do on any diet of 1000 calories or less, your body thinks you are starving (because you are). It believes you are in the middle of a famine, so it dramatically slows down metabolism which is the rate at which your body burns fuel. If you reduce your food intake by 25%, then your metabolic rate may slow down by as much as 20 to 25%. To avoid "starvation" your body automatically turns down your built-in thermostat. Like a thermostat that's been re-adjusted, your metabolic "set point" may change, causing your metabolism to remain at the lower rate. When your metabolic rate is lower, you burn calories more slowly. Just as a car at lower speeds burns less gasoline.

Remember from past dieting how you always lost the most weight in the first few weeks. As your body's metabolism starts slowing down, it begins to fight against your good intention of losing weight. This "plateau" effect is why it is so hard to continue losing weight as time rolls on.

When your body slides into this "slow down" cycle, your metabolic rate stays depressed for up to two months, even "after you start eating normally again". When you stop dieting by restricting calories and return to your (before dieting) regular eating habits, the depressed metabolic rate *ensures* rapid weight gain.

In other words, repeated dieting leads to more lowering of your metabolic rate. When you get tired of feeling hungry and go off the diet, you may gain back even more than you lost, although you eat the same amount of food as you did before you started to diet. This leads to the familiar *"Yo-Yo phenomenon"* in which dieters lose some weight, then gain it all back and then some. This can happen over and over again.

Your Body Is Not Listening

You can try explaining to your body that you are not trying to save body fat, you are trying to get rid of it, but your body is programmed not to listen. The more your food intake drops, the harder your body tries to keep from losing fat.

By nature your body resists diets. In times past, only a shortage of food could cause people to starve. Only those who could deal with a temporary period of starvation survived. Your body has a built-in mechanism to survive in the case of a shortage of food.

Natural biological mechanisms kick into action to counter starvation. First, your body turns down the metabolic "flame" to save as much body fat as possible until the starvation period is over. This body fat is your fuel reserve. Next, your body gets set to binge on the first available food.

Binges and the "Restrained-Eater" Phenomenon

Another of the body's defense mechanisms against starvation is to binge. This is an automatic mechanism. Your body cannot tell the difference from a restricted calorie diet or a journey through a desert, where the food may be scarce for a long time. Dr. Neal Barnard, a noted psychiatrist and foremost health authority, calls this the "Restrained-Eater" phenomenon.

He asks, "Does this sound familiar? You have been dieting for several days. You had a tiny breakfast, skipped lunch, and then in the evening someone brings home a carton of ice cream. A little bit won't hurt, you decide as you take a taste, and before you know it you are scraping the bottom of the carton and digging around the cracks for every last bite."

He continues, "You then feel remorse for your 'lack of willpower'. Your body disconnected your brain, in effect, in order to accomplish a predictable biological phenomenon. Your body was operating on the assumption that the food in front of you might be the only food you would have for a while, so it demanded a binge."

Frequent binges can turn into bulimia: binge eating is often followed by purging. Bulimia almost always begins with a diet and ends with a sense of shame and moral failing. It is not a moral failing. It is a natural biological consequence of dieting. So many children and teenagers are raised on meals of fatty foods that cause them to gain weight. They mistakenly think that the problem is quantity of food they eat, rather than the type of food, so they begin restricting calories. The natural result is lowered metabolic rates, cravings and binges.[4]

ANIMAL FAT AND FRIES SPELL "FAT ON YOU"

Today the American diet is loaded with meat. Meat on the average is about 65 percent fat calories.

Americans pig out on fatty French fries, onion rings, corn chips, potato chips and fat-drenched chip dips. It's no wonder we are getting fatter!

Earlier in this century our ancestors ate whole wheat bread, beans, unrefined whole cereals, vegetables, rice, and fruits. Meats were not eaten every day. They were too expensive. But today, almost everyone can afford fatty hamburgers, fried fish sandwiches, fried chicken, French fries, cheese, milk shakes, and other fatty fast foods, **and they eat it all day long.** Milk, butter, and eggs, are all loaded with fat too. All this adds up and means *"The Fat You Eat Is The Fat You Wear."*

Carbohydrates Increase Metabolism and Burn Fat

Foods from plants are the only source of complex carbohydrates. Complex carbohydrate is a scientific term for molecules made up of many sugars linked together. When you eat the starchy white insides of a potato or any other edible plant, the carbohydrate is slowly broken apart into simple sugars, which are then absorbed and used by the body. Animal foods contain little if any carbohydrate.

Again quoting Dr. Neal Barnard, "Carbohydrate-rich meals are not just low in calories. They re-adjust your hormones, which in turn boost your metabolism and speed up the burning of calories. One of these hormones is a Thyroid hormone called T4, so named because it has four iodine atoms attached. This hormone has two possible fates: It can be converted into the active form of thyroid hormone called

T3, which boosts your metabolism and keeps your body burning calories, or it can be converted to an inactive hormone, called reverse T3. When your diet is rich in carbohydrates, more of the T4 is converted to T3, and your metabolism gets a good boost. If your diet is low in carbohydrates, more of the T4 is turned into reverse T3, resulting in a slowed metabolism.

"The same thing occurs during periods of very low-calorie dieting or starvation. Less of the T4 is converted to T3 and more to the useless reverse T3. This is presumably the body's way of guarding its reserves of fat; when not much food is coming in, the body conserves fat and turns down the production of the fat-burning hormone, T3. But a diet generous in carbohydrates keeps T3 levels high and keeps the fat fires burning."[5]

Norepinephrine, a relative of adrenaline is also produced when we eat carbohydrates, increasing metabolism even more. Carbohydrates also help cue the body to stop eating. The body adjusts your appetite based on the carbohydrate content you eat. In other words, when you eat meats and fat which contain practically no carbohydrate you will eat more food. When you eat plant-food which is mostly carbohydrate your body naturally cues you to stop eating before you overeat.

Fructose, a natural sugar in fruits, may play a part in diminishing your appetite and your desire for fatty foods according to some researchers.

Fiber contains almost no calories but adds texture to foods making them more satisfying. Fiber is only found in plants. Animal foods, (red meats, chicken, fish, all dairy products, milk, cheese, eggs, and fats) contain no fiber. You need 40 to 60 grams of fiber each day which can only be obtained naturally if you eat a "Plantarian" diet.[5]

What are the Major Sources of Fat?

Guess what the most fattening foods are? Meats (and that means all flesh—including poultry and fish), most dairy products, fried foods, vegetable oils, and salad dressings. They are all loaded with fat, as high as 99%. Fat is, *surprisingly,* the most fattening nutrient of the diet of affluent western societies.

If you eat fat (animal or vegetable) it is added to your body fat with a loss of only about 3% of it's calories in the process. In contrast, if the body tries to store the energy of carbohydrates it has to chemically convert it to fat, a process which consumes nearly 25% of its calories. A small part of the fat you eat is used for energy and part is added to the fat stores you already have.

Compare rice with chicken. A one-half cup serving of rice contains 100 calories of carbohydrate. If the body tries to convert it into fat, nearly 25% of its calories are burned up in the process. Rice contains almost no fat, only one-tenth of a gram. A chicken breast, on the other hand, contains **NO** carbohydrates and nearly all the fat can easily be added to your body.

Two-thirds of a chicken breast contains about 100 calories of fat. If you eat these 100 fat-calories, only three calories may be used for energy. Theoretically, 97 calories could end up as body fat on you.[6]

A Natural Means of Weight Loss

Conventional diets call for small portions to reduce calories sufficiently. Because of this you feel hungry and deprived. It's no wonder—you're starving!

The Miracle Diet Program is based on the latest scientific research revealing that it's the **TYPE** of food *not* the **QUANTITY** that keeps you lean and healthy.

The truth is you can eat until you're satisfied and still lose weight. You'll never feel hungry or deprived again.

You say, "How is this possible?"

The Answer is *"THE MIRACLE DIET"*

All you have to do is change your fuel to a plant-centered diet and discard the old, high-fat diet.

Your metabolic thermostat will be set at a higher level which burns more calories. Also, a mild easy-to-do exercise program should be incorporated into your lifestyle because when fitness goes up, metabolism goes up. Sedentary living is not natural for humans. (Refer to Chapter 14, "Change: Making it All Work With Diet And Exercise").

For Even Faster Weight Loss

If you want to lose weight even faster use only a limited amount, if any, of finely ground flour products, such as breads, crackers, pretzels, etc. The body absorbs calories too easily when natural grains are ground into fine flours.

Eat only the following plant foods if you want to lose weight faster:

- Whole-grain cereals, whole grains like corn and brown rice, coarsely ground wheat, oats and barley, whole berries of wheat, oatmeal, commercial packaged cereals such as Wheatena, Zoom, and other less-refined hot cereals. Cold cereals like Shredded Wheat, Grapenuts, etc., are also acceptable.
- Potatoes, yams, sweet potatoes, and carrots.
- Legumes, like pinto, navy, kidney, and black beans as well as peas, string beans, lentils, split peas, and black-eyed peas.
- Yellow and green vegetables like cabbage, different types of lettuce, celery, cauliflower, broccoli, asparagus, kale, spinach, and collard greens. Tomatoes are good too.
- Various squashes, like butternut, hubbard, zucchini, acorn, spaghetti squash, summer squash, etc.
- Fruit, bananas, apples, oranges, grapefruit, pears, peaches, berries. Limit your fruit to three or less servings each day because fruit is high in simple carbohydrates (sugars).
- Fat-free rice milk and fat-free soy milk are suggested for cooking or use on cereals.

There is plenty of variety and great flavor in the various plant foods listed above. Maybe you are one of those people whose metabolism is at a lower set point from past calorie cutting and yo-yo dieting. You may need to concentrate on the list of plant foods with more bulk and less concentration of calories.

These foods can be enjoyed and relished when you learn how to use spices, herbs, and the wonderful recipes at the end of this book and THE MIRACLE DIET COOKBOOK by the same author.

Foods to Avoid To Be Lean and Healthy

For the *"Best Possible Health"* and a slim, attractive body, **avoid** the following:

- All dairy products, butter, cheese, yogurt and cow's milk. (See Chapter Seven on milk).
- All fowl, poultry, and fish. They are as high in cholesterol as red meat.
- All beef, pork and lamb. Use no red meat.
- All eggs. They are loaded with cholesterol and fat.
- All cooking oils like corn oil, canola oil, peanut and safflower oil, including olive oil.
- Severely limit or avoid avocados, nuts, seeds, olives, coconut and chocolate, also most soybean products unless they are fat free.
- Fruit juices and dried fruit are high in simple carbohydrates (sugars) and should be limited.
- Finely ground grain flours; if used at all, should be limited for faster weight loss.
- Simple carbohydrates like honey, sugar, molasses, syrup, etc., should be very limited.
- Salt should be limited to be used directly on food at the table. Use Mrs. Dash, herbs and spices instead.

A proper diet does not require you to go hungry. Always be satisfied and feel that you have eaten all you want. Plant foods (complex carbohydrates) do satisfy your hunger drive and provide your body maximum energy.

As you read on you will be more and more convinced that plant food is the proper fuel for man. As you discover the pleasure and satisfaction of eating right, you will be happy to be a "Plantarian" because you'll be attractive, lean, and enjoying the *"Best Possible Health."*

This book contains many easy menus and exciting, delicious recipes that will tickle your taste buds. The flavors will delight your senses and will make eating a rich, colorful experience!

For hundreds of additional mouth-watering recipes look for our companion book with the red cover, *"THE MIRACLE DIET COOKBOOK,"* by Earl and Ethel Updike.

Two

The Miracle
Diet Program

This book was written to give you the knowledge and the desire to change your life and become the attractive, healthy, vital, productive person you want to be.

What will happen as a result of following this program? Plenty! You'll lose excess weight. You'll enjoy boundless energy. You'll protect yourself from degenerative diseases. You'll look young well into old age. Simply stated, you'll enjoy the *"Best Possible Health!"*

That's not all. You'll do it without spending lots of money on fad diet plans, liposuction, plastic surgery, expensive cosmetics, or diet supplements. Instead you'll do it with inexpensive, enjoyable healthy foods. It is a program that can make you look and feel your physical best. What more could you possibly ask for? The price is certainly right, and you'll save up to 50 percent on your grocery bill.

The Miracle Diet

Humans are primates, and like monkeys, apes, and gorillas we should live mainly on plants. You will never see a monkey eat steak. Like our primate "cousins," we by nature, thrive best on starches. This exciting concept substitutes these basic foods (starches) as entrees for your current entrees of chicken, beef, fish, eggs, and dairy products. Meals take on a new meaning using plant foods (starches) with vegetable side dishes. Learning to eat plant food, the correct fuel for man, will produce amazing results within two-weeks.

Obesity Nearly Unknown?

In Asian countries, obesity is nearly unknown. In those countries the average diet consists mainly of the five basic starches. The Asians who remain slim for their entire lives live on a diet consisting

mostly of rice, wheat, potatoes, corn, beans, and other starchy vegetables. They *shun greasy, fatty flesh* and *dairy products.* What happens if they move to America and adopt our eating habits? They get
fat just like 71% of Americans.[1]

If you want to lose weight, do what billions of people throughout
the world do: eat the diet described in this book, a diet of plant foods.

Remember, a medium potato contains only 80 calories; a large
potato has only 150 calories; and a cup of brown rice only about 200
calories. They don't make you fat. Remember, what makes you fat is
the animal toppings you ladle on: the butter, sour cream, or a 100%
fat dressing squeezed from plants. *We call it margarine!*

The Standard American Diet is Hazardous to Your Health

The modern American diet is made up mainly of animal food
loaded with cholesterol and fats, as well as too many salts, sugars,
super-refined foods, food additives, added vegetable fats, concentrated chemical poisons, and drugs given to livestock.

A large proportion of American adults are overweight and suffer
from unnecessary degenerative diseases. As a result, medical costs
were 14% of Gross National Product in 1992 and rising rapidly.
Even those who are healthy, bear the burden by paying rising insurance rates and higher taxes to fund costly medical welfare programs.

It doesn't have to be this way. A growing number of health professionals are advocating that Americans change to a plant-based
diet for their *"Best Possible Health."* Media reporters are beginning to talk about a plant-centered diet. However, in spite of this exploding scientific knowledge, the majority of Americans continue to
get most of their calories from rich animal foods like chicken, fish,
meat, milk, cheese, ice cream, cottage cheese, sour cream, eggs,
lunch meats, and other products derived from animals. Despite this
trend, a quiet revolution is beginning.

**Healthy people have been eating a Plantarian diet for
centuries.** The Bible records that 2500 years ago, Daniel said to the
commander of the officials, *"Give us nothing but vegetables to eat and
water to drink. Then compare our appearance with that of the young
men who eat the royal food, and treat your servants in accordance
with what you see. So he agreed to this and tested them for ten days.*

At the end of ten days they looked healthier and better nourished than any of the young men who ate the royal food. So the guard took away their choice food and the wine they were to drink and gave them vegetables instead."
                    Daniel 1 The Bible, New International Version (1984)

Where Do You Get Your Protein?

Amazingly the *best* possible food sources for protein are *grains, vegetables, legumes (beans, peas, lentils),* and *fruits* in an unrefined, minimally processed form.[2] Animal food is **not** the best source of protein. It is high in fat, contains little carbohydrate and does not provide the right proportions of nutrients for energy and health. This is not what most Americans have been taught since childhood.

While we're at it, let's explore another myth. Accurate estimates of adult human needs show that as little as 2.5 percent of our daily calorie intake must come from protein. This small amount of protein equals about 20 grams (two-thirds of an ounce) for an adult man.

The World Health Organization (WHO) has established a higher minimum daily requirement for protein, at about five percent of the daily caloric intake. Studies show that many populations have lived in excellent health on less than 5 percent protein. WHO has set pregnancy protein requirements at 6 percent, and lactation requirements at 6.7 percent of daily calorie intake.

What Does That Mean In Real Terms?

A working man eating 3,000 calories a day at 5 percent protein needs only 150 of those calories as protein. With each gram of protein amounting to 4 calories, this would represent only 37 grams of protein. The average woman who consumes 2,300 calories daily needs only 29 grams of protein, according to WHO.

These minimum requirements provide a large margin of safety in the event some people might have greater protein needs. This small quantity of protein is almost impossible to avoid if you eat enough food to satisfy your hunger.[3]

Dr. John McDougall says, "Excess amounts of proteins (especially of animal proteins) cause change in kidney activity, resulting in large losses of calcium from the body. Experimental studies show that protein levels commonly consumed by Americans (90 grams and more—over 15 percent of the calories) will cause more calcium to be lost from the body than can be absorbed from the gut, even when the person is consuming very high levels of calcium. This is why populations around the world that eat rich diets loaded with animal proteins (as in the United States, England, Israel, Finland, Sweden, etc.) have high rates of osteoporosis, while people in countries that consume small amounts of animal proteins (including dairy foods), such as those living in Asian and African countries, have strong bones and little osteoporosis."[4]

Can You Get Enough Protein From Plants?

Yes! Plant food supplies plenty of protein. For example, 3,000 calories of white potatoes alone provide 80 grams of excellent protein; the same amount of rice would supply 60 grams of quality protein.[5]

How good is the protein provided by plants? The building blocks of proteins are the amino acids. Varied combinations among the twenty or so amino acids form the proteins found in humans and all other living creatures. Surprisingly enough, *all* plant foods contain all twenty or so amino acids, as do animal foods. However, the amount of each amino acid that is present varies in different foods. Humans and animals can synthesize some of the needed amino acids, but others must be obtained from food. The amino acids that cannot be synthesized and which must be obtained from food are known as essential amino acids. Humans require eight and some theorize nine essential amino acids. Plants provide all twenty or so amino acids, including the eight or nine essential ones we need.

Scientific studies over the past forty years clearly demonstrate that a starch-centered diet supplemented with additional vegetables and fruits is an excellent protein source and the foundation for the best possible nutrition.[6]

Are Plant Proteins Complete?

Some believe plants provide only incomplete protein. This misconception dates back to 1914, when Osborn and Mendel studied the protein requirements of rats. This early study was later proved wrong. Over forty years have gone by since this early study was proved false, yet this gross error continues to be perpetuated. As a result, people continue to eat animal flesh and animal by-products on a false premise.[7]

Our nutritional needs are a lot different from those of rats. If they were the same, human mother's milk would be unhealthy for babies because the protein of rat's milk is "ten times more concentrated than human mother's milk."[8] **Mother's milk contains** roughly **5 percent protein.** We know that the greatest need of protein is in the first year of life. This indicates that only a small amount of protein is needed later in life. Certainly much less than the 20–25% protein being consumed in the standard American diet.

Many mothers bottle-feed their babies with cow's milk. Whole cow's milk contains 21 percent protein, while 2 percent (low-fat) milk contains 26 percent protein—over five times more than needed. Many scientists now agree that this excessive protein intake throughout life is responsible for epidemic osteoporosis in countries where dairy products and animals are the major source of calories.[9]

The Amino Acid Myth

Experimenting on humans to determine the amino acid requirements of man, William Rose in 1952 proved that even single vegetable foods contain more than enough of all the amino acids essential for humans. Many other researchers have measured the capacity of plant foods to satisfy protein needs. The results of these studies show that strong, healthy children and adults thrive on diets based on single or combined starches.

It is important to know that any single starch, such as potatoes, brown rice, corn, beans, or grains, can supply all the needed energy and essential amino acid requirements.[10]

Are We Destined To Be Sick?

According to many scientific authorities, if Americans had followed *"The Miracle Diet"* since childhood, very few of us would suffer from major diseases such as atherosclerosis, heart disease, high blood pressure, stroke, diabetes, diet-related cancers, osteoporosis, urinary disease, arthritis, or obesity. Few of us would be bothered by minor, yet painful, diseases such as diverticulitis, hiatus hernia, appendicitis, gallstones, hemorrhoids, kidney stones, varicose veins, and constipation, which are associated with the low-fiber, high-fat, cholesterol-laden animal food we eat .[11]

In societies where people follow the principles of *"The Miracle Diet,"* these diseases essentially do not exist. In China, people eat approximately 80 percent complex carbohydrates, 10 percent fat, and 10 percent protein, the very combination contained in a variety of grains, legumes, vegetables, and fruits. The Chinese eat very little flesh or animal food of any kind, and dairy products are virtually unknown. The main source of calories is starches—rice, potatoes, beans, corn wheat, barley, oats, and other grains, supplemented with vegetables and fruits.[12–17]

In stark contrast America eats approximately 45 percent of total calories in fat, 20 percent in protein, and 25 percent in (simple refined) carbohydrates. Only about 10 percent complex carbohydrates. In addition, we eat from 300 to 1000 milligrams of cholesterol each day, all of which comes from animal flesh and other animal products.

The bulk of our calories comes from animal flesh (meat, fish, and fowl), other animal foods (milk, cheese, ice cream, cottage cheese, sour cream, butter, eggs, and so on), and added vegetable fats (margarine, cooking oils, shortening, and salad dressings).

Where Is The Fiber?

Fat content isn't the only problem. *Animal foods contain no fiber,* which is absolutely necessary to maintain proper health. Animal foods are the only foods that contain cholesterol, which is the basic cause of atherosclerosis, the destruction of the inner lining of the arteries and blood vessels. Atherosclerosis leads to heart attacks, strokes, aneurysms, kidney diseases, and many other degenerative conditions.

Is Sugar the Culprit?

Is it any wonder why so few of us are within the ideal weight range? Too many people blame sugar. The average American does eat 135 pounds of sugar each year, but sugar isn't the major cause of obesity. Sugar should, in fact, be limited because it contains no fiber and consists only of empty calories that take the place of complex carbohydrates. However, the real cause of obesity is excessive fat, which comes from animal products and added vegetable fats. Fats seem to enhance salty and sugary tastes. Perhaps that's why we are tempted to consume nearly 50 percent of our total calories as fat.[18]

Happiness Is Our Goal

We have been taught from childhood that happiness is our goal in this life. It is much more difficult to be happy when we or those we love are sick and broken down with disease.

Today medical science is proving the need for more and more plant food in our diet if we want to enjoy optimal health and long life.

On this page, you will see clearly the very low fat content of plant foods. Plants contain plenty of protein, no cholesterol and are rich in needed fiber.

Low Fat: Examples of Plants, Starches, Vegetables, Fruit

Percentage of Calories:

	% Protein	% Fat	Cholesterol
Apple	trace	trace	0
Beans (pinto)	23%	3%	0
Beans (lima)	25%	3%	0
Barley	9%	3%	0
Broccoli	44%	6%	0
Cabbage	26%	trace	0
Carrots	13%	trace	0
Cauliflower	32%	trace	0
Celery	20%	trace	0
Corn (ear)	14%	10%	0
Oranges	7%	trace	0
Oatmeal	17%	12%	0
Pears	4%	9%	0
Peas (green, frozen)	26%	trace	0
Potatoes	9%	trace	0
Rice (brown)	9%	4%	0
Spaghetti (white, cooked)	15%	5%	0
Sweet Potatoes	7%	trace	0
Whole wheat flour	16%	5%	0

Only animal foods contain cholesterol. They are much too high in protein. They contain no fiber and are loaded with saturated fat that your body makes into more cholesterol.

High Fat: Examples of Animal Foods Which Must Be Severely Limited If You Want To Be Lean and Healthy[19]

Percentage of Calories:

	% Protein	% Fat	Cholesterol
Beef (chuck roast) 3 oz.	27%	72%	87 mg.
Butter, 1/2 cup	0%	100%	247 mg.
Cheddar Cheese, 1 oz.	24%	73%	30 mg.
Chicken (breast, baked, no skin) 3 oz	77%	19%	73 mg.
Cottage Cheese (regular 4%) 1 cup	48%	38%	34 mg.
Cottage Cheese (low-fat 2%) 1 cup	60%	18%	19 mg.
Egg, one	30%	66%	274 mg.
Lamb Loin (broiled) 2.8 oz.	37%	61%	78 mg.
Milk (whole 3.3%) 1 cup	21%	48%	33 mg.
Milk (low-fat 2%) 1 cup	26%	38%	18 mg.
Pork loin (broiled) 3.1 oz.	35%	62%	84 mg.
Salmon (baked) 3 oz.	60%	32%	60 mg.
Tuna (canned in oil) 3 oz.	58%	38%	55 mg.
Tuna (canned in water) 3 oz.	89%	7%	48 mg.
Turkey (roasted) 3 oz.	57%	35%	45 mg.

Ideal Weight

This weight chart indicates Dr. Walter Kempner's evaluation of reasonable adult weight in proportion to height. (Bulletin of the Kempner Foundation, Durham, N.C. 4:47, 1972.)

Women (fully dressed)		Men (fully dressed)	
Height	Weight in Pounds	Height	Weight in Pounds
4'11".	91	5'2".	110
5'	94	5'3".	115
5'1".	97	5'4".	120
5'2".	100	5'5".	125
5'3".	104	5'6".	130
5'4".	108	5'7".	135
5'5".	112	5'8".	140
5'6".	117	5'9".	145
5'7".	122	5'10".	150
5'8".	127	5'11".	155
5'9".	132	6'	160
5'10".	137	6'1".	165
5'11".	142	6'2".	170
6'	147	6'3".	175
		6'4".	180
		6'5".	185

Compared to average weights in the Western world, these numbers seem low. But if you change to a "Plantarian" diet, you will find they are actually attainable.[20]

Three

Put Prevention First

You, personally, are the solution to the national health care crisis.

Doctors, nurses, hospitals, clinics, insurance companies or government programs cannot give you health. Only you can give yourself and your family health by changing your lifestyle and the type of food you eat.

According to the US Surgeon General's Report on Nutrition and Health (1988), ***most illness in America are caused by diet and lifestyle practices and therefore are preventable.***

Prevention Is NOT Early Detection and Treatment

Heart disease, stroke, breast cancer, prostate cancer, colon cancer, adult diabetes, osteoporosis, high blood pressure, obesity and many other preventable diseases cause untold pain, misery and up to 80% of all deaths in America each year.

Prevention comes from following a "Plantarian" starch-based diet: avoiding tobacco, alcohol and drugs gives an extra cushion of protection. Include regular exercise such as walking. Learning to relax and keeping a positive attitude also help prevent disease.

Over 3 billion people worldwide eat a plant-centered diet, with little added fat, no milk products after weaning and very little animal foods. These people are comparatively free of heart disease, stroke, breast cancer, prostate cancer, colon cancer, diabetes, obesity, osteoporosis, arthritis and multiple sclerosis.

In the United States however, we spend about 1 trillion dollars a year on health care and costs may soon amount to 20% of the Gross National Product. This crisis could overwhelm our entire financial system.

As has been pointed out before, human beings are primates along with the apes, gorillas, and monkeys (see any dictionary). Primates are primarily herbivores (plant eaters or Plantarians). Most will only eat flesh if plant foods are unavailable.

Animal food and high fat are the wrong fuel for humans, as wrong as using diesel fuel in a gasoline engine which will destroy the engine. It is clear from worldwide epidemiological studies and a consensus of medical scientists that plant food should be our major source of calories for optimum health. A plant-centered diet is the correct fuel for man.

The "New Four Food Groups"

The **"New Four Food Groups"** were introduced to the world in 1991 by the Physicians Committee for Responsible Medicine, a large body of medical doctors. They declare that grain, legumes, vegetables, and fruit are the food (fuel) for man. Meat, chicken, fish, eggs and dairy products are not needed in our diet.

Their message is: To prevent debilitating and killer degenerative diseases we must immediately change to a **plant-based** intake of calories and stop adding vegetable fat and oils to our diet.

A growing number of nurses, medical doctors, scientists, and other health professionals are adopting a plant-centered food program for the *"Best Possible Health."* The American people are starting to recognize that an animal-based diet is making them fat, sick, and tired. By following the program in this book you will have all the tools you need to become more attractive and have the *"Best Possible Health."*

The official Food Guide Pyramid, adopted in 1992 by the USDA and the Department of Health and Human Services, is a step in the right direction and demonstrates that plant food (whole grains-vegetables-legumes-fruit) is the foundation of a balanced diet. The pyramid shows that 85% of calories daily should be derived from plants, only about 8% from animal products and only about 3.5% from added fat.

Even though the USDA Pyramid is far superior to the old "Basic Four Food Groups" (1956 to 1992), it falls far short of the *"Best*

Possible Health" because it includes meat, chicken, fish, eggs and milk products.

You Can Help!

Call or write your Congressional Representatives. You are welcome to copy and send them the seven point solution that follows.

Talk to your state legislators and school board members about changing the laws in your state and school district concerning the high fat content and large amount of animal food in school lunches. The food now being served is not only making children fat, it is making sure that over half of these kids will eventually die of heart disease, some at very early ages. Twenty-five percent will suffer and die of cancer mostly because of the food they learned to eat at school.

The Solution to the Health Care Crisis
Is Education About Prevention

1. *Governments and schools must begin an all-out media blitz and educational programs to promote and teach that plant food must be the foundation of our daily diet.*

2. *Total fat intake must be drastically reduced to 10% of daily calories to prevent and reverse degenerative diseases.*

3. *Fiber must be increased from 10 grams per day to between 40-60 grams per day.*

4. *Encourage health insurance companies to develop policies that have premiums based upon a person's controlable risk factors which can be determined by weight, blood pressure and blood cholesterol levels. These can be easily measured. Wellness saves everyone money. Health care costs could be cut in half within one year.*

5. *Change is EASY when we once learn which foods provide the proper fuel and their direct effect on our long and short term health. Teach the relationship between food and health from kindergarten through college.*

6. *The Chinese have a slogan—"PUT PREVENTION FIRST." Let's adapt an old American adage "Why Fix It If It Ain't Broke" and say, "WHY FIX IT WHEN IT CAN BE PREVENTED."*

7. *Only a PREVENTION program will solve the health care crisis in America.*

Four

Herbivores versus Carnivores

Contrary to popular belief, human bodies resemble those of herbivores (plant eaters), **NOT** carnivores (animal eaters).[1] Based upon physical comparison, one would have a difficult time making a case for humans being carnivores in any way. On the other hand, it can easily be shown that human bodies are made like those of other known herbivores.[2–6] For example:

Human bodies resemble those of apes, chimpanzees, monkeys, and gorillas[7] more closely than those of any other animal in creation. Primates are almost exclusively herbivores.

1. Humans, like all herbivores, have flat, back molar teeth for grinding plant food. Carnivores have sharp teeth all the way to the back of their mouths for ripping and tearing flesh.

2. Carnivores have livers that excrete nearly 100 percent of all cholesterol from the flesh they eat. Herbivores, including humans, have livers with a limited capacity to excrete excess cholesterol. If humans and other herbivores eat more cholesterol than their livers can excrete, the retained cholesterol and saturated fat cause disease and death.

3. Humans have a long, convoluted gut like that of other herbivores to digest plant food. Carnivores, on the other hand, have a very short gut for the digestion of flesh.[8]

4. Humans have enzymes in their intestines that digest complex carbohydrates; carnivores do not have these enzymes.

5. Humans have alpha amylase, an enzyme in saliva that digests complex carbohydrates. This enzyme is not present in carnivores.

6. Humans and most plant-eating animals have well-developed salivary glands, alkaline saliva, and secrete a starch-splitting en-

zyme in the saliva known as ptyalin. Carnivores have small salivary glands with acid saliva and no ptyalin.

7. Carnivores have a 20 times higher concentration of hydrochloric acid in their stomachs than humans or other herbivores.

8. Carnivores have claws. Humans and herbivores have no claws.

Similarities and Differences Between Carnivores, Herbivores and Man[9] by Dr. Marc Sorenson		
Carnivores	**Herbivores**	**Man**
Has claws	**NO** claws	**NO** claws
Has sharp pointed front teeth	**NO** sharp pointed front teeth	**NO** sharp pointed front teeth
NO flat back molar teeth	Has flat back molar teeth	Has flat back molar teeth
NO pores on skin	Pores on skin	Pores on skin
Small salivary glands	Well-developed salivary glands	Well-developed salivary glands
Acid saliva	Alkaline saliva	Alkaline saliva
NO ptyalin in saliva	Ptyalin in saliva	Ptyalin in saliva
Much hydrochloric acid in stomach	Hydrochloric acid in stomach 1/20th as strong as meat eaters	Hydrochloric acid in stomach 1/20th as strong as meat eaters
Short intestinal tract— 3 times trunk length	Long intestinal tract— 10 to 12 times trunk length	Long intestinal tract— 12 times trunk length

Just a sidelight to further illustrate the difference between herbivores and carnivores; most herbivores, including humans, sip water and sweat through their pores while most carnivores lap water and sweat through their tongues.

The only way we humans resemble carnivores in affluent America and in the Western world, is that we eat like carnivores!

Five

Cholesterol
Kills

Approximately two million people die in the United States each year. Half of all those deaths (over a million people!) die of coronary heart or artery disease. In fact, the number-one killer in the United States since 1900 has been cardio-vascular disease with one exception (1918). Coronary heart-artery disease has become a modern-day plague, affecting all affluent, animal-eating nations.

"Total cardiovascular disease" will cost Americans an estimated 138 billion in 1995 for medical costs and disability. Nearly one out of three Americans have been diagnosed with artery disease. If you eat animal food as your main source of calories, chances are you will develop the disease.[1]

This year as many as 1.5 million Americans will have a heart attack, and more than one-third of them will die. Many will be under the age of forty.

Strokes killed 149,200 people in this country in 1987 and ranked as our nation's third largest cause of death, behind heart attack and cancer. Approximately 500,000 people suffer strokes each year, and nearly 30 percent are under the age sixty-five.

Almost all Americans have blood cholesterol values higher than 150 mg/percent, making them subject to heart-artery diseases.

There were an estimated 468,000 bypass surgeries done in the United States in 1992 at an estimated cost of $23 billion.[2] These surgeries stop chest pain in about 90 percent of the cases, but large-scale studies show that most are not necessary to save life.

There is a straight-line correlation between the amount of animal food we eat and deaths from heart-artery disease—the more animal food and cholesterol, the higher the incidence. The more animal food and cholesterol, the greater the risk of disability and death from heart-artery disease. *(Figure 1)*

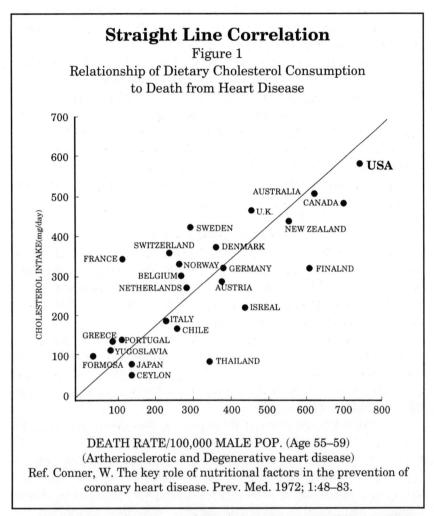

Straight Line Correlation
Figure 1
Relationship of Dietary Cholesterol Consumption
to Death from Heart Disease

DEATH RATE/100,000 MALE POP. (Age 55–59)
(Artheriosclerotic and Degenerative heart disease)
Ref. Conner, W. The key role of nutritional factors in the prevention of
coronary heart disease. Prev. Med. 1972; 1:48–83.

Heart-artery disease, or atherosclerosis, causes rotten arteries. It literally destroys blood vessels from the inside out, and progresses each day as you eat animal food. You don't have nerve endings on the inside of your arteries, so you can't feel the open, festering sores and wounds that grow there.

As time goes on, the body tries to cover up the sores created by cholesterol and fat. First, fatty streaks and deposits occur. Then the arteries develop mounds full of fat, cholesterol, and other material. These are called plaques. As this condition progresses, the entire artery becomes weak and deteriorated.[3-5]

Atherosclerosis is nearly 100-percent preventable. To immunize yourself against heart-artery disease, you must keep your cholesterol level at 150 mg/percent or less for the rest of your life, regardless of your present age. Studies, including the on-going forty-year Framingham Study, have established this "immunity level."

When a plantarian diet is your major source of calories, it is relatively easy to keep your cholesterol at 150 mg/percent or less, virtually guaranteeing immunity from heart-artery disease. *Because there is no cholesterol in any plant food.*

What is Cholesterol?

Dr. Julian Whitaker says, "Cholesterol itself is not a fat but a waxy non-caloric substance carried in the bloodstream along with fat. It is essential to life and necessary for the production of sex hormones and adrenal hormones, as well as vitamin D. It is also necessary for the synthesis of bile for digestion.

"The body produces all of the cholesterol it needs for these functions, and if you did not eat any cholesterol, your blood level would stay at the very safe 150 mg. (average) percent range. There is never a need to eat any cholesterol. Cholesterol is not a nutrient and ingestion of it can only harm you."

Dr. Whitaker states that "When you eat cholesterol, it enters the body and adds to the blood cholesterol level, elevating it from the safe range of 150 to the very high ranges found in the American population. Numerous studies, as far back as the late '50s and early '60s demonstrated that cholesterol and fat (primarily saturated fat, found in animal foods) markedly elevate the blood cholesterol level."[6]

Dr. John McDougall reveals that "When we eat the diet commonly consumed by people of affluent societies, we take in an additional 500 to 1000 milligrams of cholesterol a day, all of which comes from animal flesh and other animal products. Approximately half of the amount consumed is absorbed into the body. Plants do not make or contain cholesterol."[7]

The Chicken and Fish Myth

Chicken and fish have somehow gained the reputation of being health foods. Ironically, their cholesterol content is virtually the same as that of red meats (beef, pork, lamb and veal).

One of the latest studies shows that fish and chicken contain more cholesterol than beef. The Standard Dietitian's Reference Guide, "Food Values of Portions Commonly Used", states on page 136 that a 3.5 oz. serving of lean ground beef has 84 mg. of cholesterol. Now everybody knows that red meat is bad news, but lets look at chicken, page 160, light meat without skin, roasted, 3.5 oz. serving holds 85 mg. of cholesterol. Chicken has virtually the same amount of cholesterol as beef. A 3.5 oz. serving of fish contains about the same amount.

Let's look more closely at cholesterol and *you* on a meal to meal basis. Every time *you* eat 100 mg. (4oz.) of beef, chicken, or fish, it raises your blood cholesterol about 5 points. There is some variation from one person to another. For instance, if you consume 400 to 600 mg. of cholesterol daily, as most Americans do, it is responsible for adding from 20 to 30 points to your cholesterol level. This can eventually spell disease and death for up to 80% of all Americans.

How unfortunate that we have been given incorrect information by most nutritionists and physicians who have advised us *"just to cut down on beef"* and to *"eat fish and chicken instead,"* to lower our cholesterol levels. **All flesh (that is all animals and animal by-products) contain cholesterol. Eat it, and you risk heart disease.**

Get the Saturated Fat Out

Virtually all animal foods contain cholesterol but there's something else that's even worse—saturated fat. Most of the fat from animals is saturated fat. It's the worst kind of fat because saturated fat stimulates your liver to make additional cholesterol.[8-9]

Can anyone compensate for previous bad habits? Yes! Within two days of the time you stop eating animal foods and fat, your body begins to heal itself. Cholesterol and fat, both irritants, are gone from your fuel, and the festering sores inside your blood vessels begin the healing process.

Recent double-blind studies on humans prove that not only is atherosclerosis *caused* by what we eat, but it can be *reversed*.[9]

Proof Positive!
Heart Disease Can Be Reversed

Dr. Dean Ornish of the University of California at San Francisco medical school and a team of ten researchers conducted a landmark study on reversing heart disease with diet alone. No drugs were used. Dr. Ornish described the entire program in his book, *Dr. Ornish's Program for Reversing Heart Disease* (Random House, 1990).

The forty-eight participants in the study were of various ages (the oldest was 75), and all had severe heart disease (atherosclerosis). They were divided into two groups.

Control Group

The control group followed the American Heart Association diet consisting of 30 percent of total calories from fat and 300 milligrams of cholesterol daily.

Experimental Group

The experimental group was allowed only 10 percent of total calories as fat and 5 milligrams of cholesterol daily. Other than one cup of non-fat milk or yogurt per day and a few egg whites for cooking, the experimental group was allowed no animal products. Their entire calorie intake basically came from plant food—starches, grains, beans, vegetables, and fruit.

Results of the Study

At the end of one year, most of the experimental group on the plant diet reported their chest pains had virtually disappeared. Arterial clogging had reversed in 82 percent of the patients. Those who were the sickest at the beginning of the program showed the most improvement. Patients in the *Control Group* on the standard American Heart Association regimen all reported increased chest pain and their arterial blockage worsened.

In addition to reversing heart disease, the average weight loss on the plant-food group was 28 pounds. One person lost 100 pounds.

All of the participants in Dr. Ornish's experimental group said they would continue eating plant food because they liked it and felt better. A 75-year-old man in the group who could barely walk across the street without chest pains when he joined the program said that afterward he could hike for hours in the mountains.[10-13]

Fifty percent of Americans who die each year are poisoned by cholesterol and saturated fat that is consumed in their diet. The dictionary definition of poison is, "A substance causing illness or death when eaten, drunk, or absorbed even in relatively small quantities" (Webster's New World Dictionary).

Cholesterol is almost impossible to break down or destroy, so the only way the body can get rid of it is to excrete it through the liver, down the bile duct, into the bowel, and out of the body.

Your liver has a very limited capacity to excrete cholesterol. If you eat food that contains cholesterol, there is a net accumulation. The accumulation has to be stored in the artery walls and the body tissues. In time, the deposits become large. It may take up to five years on a cholesterol-free diet to get rid of the accumulation.[14]

Atherosclerosis Starts Early in Life

On the standard American diet signs of artery disease begin to show up in nine-month-old babies. By the age of three, a child begins to develop fatty streaks inside the artery walls. As most children reach adolescence, artery disease is well established.[15]

An interesting study was done during the Korean War. Three hundred American soldiers who had been killed in battle were autopsied. When researchers examined the soldiers' heart arteries, they found that 77 percent had atherosclerosis, or what is commonly known as "hardening of the arteries." Scar tissue was well developed, and it had become more than just fat deposits. Of the three hundred soldiers, eight had 95 percent or greater closure of at least one of their main heart arteries. In other words, they had suffered or were about to suffer a heart attack.

The most significant and shocking part of this study was the average age of these three hundred soldiers was twenty-two years![16] According to accepted medical standards, these were supposedly some of our best-conditioned men, yet they suffered an epidemic of disease.

By comparison autopsy studies on native Korean soldiers showed no evidence of early atherosclerosis. They were protected from the ravages of atherosclerosis by their plant-centered diet, low in fat and virtually devoid of cholesterol.

Even teenagers and those in their twenties sometimes suffer strokes and heart attacks, and some college athletes have died while competing or practicing.

We see much more evidence of heart attacks and strokes among those in their thirties than we used to see in this age group in past years. Heart-artery disease now manifests itself in the forties and fifties when people start to expect heart attacks. From age 60 on up, heart disease becomes the *"accepted way to die."* And here's the greatest tragedy: *coronary artery disease is nearly 100 percent preventable.*[17]

If you don't believe that heart-artery disease is preventable, take a look around the world. Cultures that eat mostly plant foods are virtually immune from heart disease. One of the best examples is the Japanese.

Traditional Japanese eat mounds of rice with fruits and vegetables and a little fish. Many Japanese smoke heavily, at about twice the U.S. rate. Their highly competitive careers and schooling put them under great physical and emotional stress. They have twice as much pollution as we do. Yet with all these traditional risk factors, the Japanese death rate from heart disease is one-tenth ours. And don't chalk it up to heredity. When the Japanese move to America and begin eating our rich animal foods, within one generation they suffer from heart-artery disease just as much as we do.

What About Heredity?

Do genes play a role? With half of our population dying of heart disease, it's hard to find any family that has escaped. But the fact that heart-artery disease strikes many families does not in any way indicate that it is an inherited disease.

If heart disease was proven to be inherited, then its incidence would be more or less constant. This is definitely the case with other proven inherited diseases, such as cystic fibrosis, Down's syndrome, hemophilia, and muscular dystrophy. These diseases are all transmitted by a gene mutation and are easily traceable within families. The incidence of these diseases is more or less constant from culture to culture.[18-19]

Heart-artery disease does not follow that pattern. For instance, as cited earlier, the Japanese suffer very little from heart disease in Japan. But when they migrate to America and adopt the American lifestyle and diet, within one generation their rate of heart-artery disease skyrockets tenfold, equaling what other Americans suffer. If heart disease were primarily an inherited disease, the protection afforded the Japanese in Japan would migrate with them to this country.

Obviously, several factors contribute to progressive atherosclerosis and heart disease. We can't control genetics, but we can control plenty of factors. The rich foods we eat, high blood pressure, obesity, cigarette smoking, inactive living, and amount of exercise are all within our control.[20]

What Part Does Stress Play?

So much has been written and discussed about stress as a factor in the development of heart-artery disease, that a great many people believe it is the only cause of the disease. Stress may tip the scale in certain cases, but it is a lifetime diet of high-cholesterol and high-fat animal food that irritates the inner lining of the arteries and causes deterioration of the blood vessels. Many researchers, in fact, feel that the role of stress is very much overrated.[21]

Let's take a look at the Japanese again as examples of what factors play the biggest role in heart disease. The Japanese usually live in a very crowded, stressful environment. They are driven by extreme competitiveness and a desire to excel. Yet with all of this drive to succeed, their rate of heart-artery disease is about one-tenth of what it is in America. Only when they change their diets do their heart disease risks increase.[22]

Another glaring example is the extreme stress upon the civilian population of Western Europe during both World War I and World War II. Studies show clearly that instead of the rate of heart-artery disease going up, it fell dramatically. Plaques in the arteries of people in their forties, fifties, sixties, and even eighties began to dissolve. The incidence of death from heart-artery disease fell so radically during both wars that the medical researchers in Western Europe began to examine it.[23]

This dramatic decrease in atherosclerosis resulted from the drastic reduction in the rich animal foods, full of cholesterol and fat, that were taken away from the civilian population during rationing. This dramatic drop in the death rate of heart-artery disease is one of the best examples for scientists world-wide to prove that atherosclerosis can and will reverse when people stop eating animals and animal by-products. Unfortunately, when rationing ended, so did freedom from heart disease. Within a few years after each war ended, heart-artery disease rates were back to normal.[24]

What About Pollution?

Clean air and clean water are important—but dirty water and air have not been proven to cause heart disease. The chemicals in the soil and those sprayed on the crops are not what we want in our environment; neither are the antibiotics and drugs that are injected into animals and fowls. But these are not the primary causes of heart-artery problems. Cholesterol and fat *have been proven to cause heart disease*.[25] A clean environment is needed, but we know the *primary* cause of heart-artery disease is animal food and fat.

Should You Be Last On The Food Chain?

When you eat animals and animal by-products you are the last on the food chain. When you eat animals and animal by-products you get in, the most concentrated form possible, all of the chemicals, hormones, and pollutants the animals ate. The least concentrated toxins are in root vegetables, grains, legumes, fruits, and leafy vegetables.[26] That alone should convince you to stop eating flesh and animal by-products as your main source of calories.

Is Impotence Caused by Eating Animal Foods?

Yes! According to researchers in France who examined 440 impotent men and found that the risk factors for impotence is the same as for heart disease. By age sixty-five, one out of four men is impotent. Just as plaques form in the coronary arteries causing heart attacks, plaques form in the arteries to the genitals causing impotence.

- Eating animal foods that contain high cholesterol and saturated fat causes plaques to form in arteries throughout the entire body.
- Fatty diets are a major cause of diabetes, which also can lead to impotence by accelerating atherosclerosis.
- Meat, dairy, eggs and other animal foods also contribute to high blood pressure which can cause atherosclerosis and in turn impotence.

Millions of Men Are Impotent

Eminent scientists have reported that approximately 10 million men in America are impotent. Impotence is defined as the consistent inability to achieve or sustain an erection sufficient for sexual intercourse.

The incidence of impotence increases with age. At age forty only 2% of men are affected. This increases to 25% by the early to mid-sixties.

Fears, such as performance anxiety, cause some men to experience psychogenic impotence (the problem being all in the man's mind) but this could not account for the unbelievable loss of function experienced by so many men as they age.

Doctors are starting to realize that most problems of impotence have a *physical cause* and that cause is primarily diet-related, not mental.

Many medical doctors now agree that the most common reason for failure to achieve an adequate erection is hardening of the arteries (atherosclerosis) to the penis. This is caused by a high-fat, high cholesterol, animal-based diet. Blockage of blood vessels may account for 80 percent of impotence suffered by men in affluent America.

An Ounce of Prevention

Plantarianism should appeal to all men who want to protect their sexual drive throughout life. The threat of impotence, ***even early in life,*** should motivate all men (and women too) to change to a plant-based eating plan.[27]

Six

Fats:
The Dreaded Enemy

Until the middle of the 20th century, most of the fats Americans ate came from animals. Before World War II, housewives saved the bacon and fat drippings for cooking or used lard or butter. Animal foods were basically the only source of added fat in the diet.

Vegetable oils and fats are a relatively new innovation and they too contribute to an already serious health problem. People seem to think that if fats come from vegetables they are "okay." As a result, our fat intake as a nation has dramatically increased.

The problem with vegetable oil comes when it is extracted from the vegetable. When corn, cotton seeds, soybeans, peanuts, and other plants are squeezed to produce oil, the other important and essential parts of the plant, such as fiber, protein, complex carbohydrates, vitamins, and minerals, are removed. The final product is 100 percent fat. And just like animal fat it overburdens the body and is the leading cause of obesity, diabetes, high blood pressure, some cancers, and many other degenerative diseases.[1]

Fats are divided into four general groups, based on their physical and chemical makeup:

1. **Saturated fats** come mostly from animals, such as beef, pork, lamb, chicken, eggs, and dairy products. Certain plant products: coconut, coconut oil, chocolate, cocoa butter, palm oil, vegetable shortening, and margarine are also high in saturated fat. These fats are usually solid at room temperature.

2. **Monounsaturated fats** are found in olives and olive oil. They are liquid at room temperature.

3. **Polyunsaturated fats** are abundant in vegetables and grains. These fats are most often fluid at room temperature. Examples: corn oil like Mazola, vegetable oil like Wesson, or Canola oil.

4. **Hydrogenated fats and oils** are produced by adding hydrogen to vegetable oils to make a more saturated product that is mostly solid at room temperature. Examples: vegetable shortenings like Crisco.

When you get right down to it, there isn't much difference. They all make you fat and can cause disease and death.

Here's why. Each gram of fat contains nine calories, compared to four calories in a gram of carbohydrate or protein. Simply stated, there are more than two times as many calories in fat as in carbohydrate or protein. There's another serious problem associated with fats as I've mentioned; our livers make cholesterol out of saturated fats.

The calories in fat are so concentrated that they take up much less space in your stomach; therefore you don't feel full, even though you have eaten foods containing many calories.[2]

Most of the fat Americans eat is from animal foods. But we also get a lot of vegetable fat from margarine and salad dressing, which are nearly 100 percent fat. On top of all that, we add vegetable and animal fats to the vegetables we cook. All added vegetable fats contain more saturated fat than you should have in your body. Most cakes, pies, and cookies contain about 50 percent of their calories in fat; many rich pastries contain much higher amounts of fat calories. Beware of these vegetable fats, the worst being tropical oils.

Many commercial baked goods contain highly saturated vegetable fats, palm kernel oil (86 percent saturated fat), and/or coconut oil (92 percent saturated fat). Avoid these tropical oils completely. In many cases these baked foods contain saturated animal fats, too. Milk chocolate contains more than 50 percent fat, both saturated and unsaturated. The average chocolate bar contains between 13 and 20 grams of fat: 180 calories from fat alone. As a matter of fact, most commercial products—baked, canned, frozen, cooked, processed—contain a high percentage of fat.[3]

There Is a Simple Solution to Obesity

The simple solution to our epidemic obesity is not chronic dieting. Instead, the answer lies in eating the foods nature has given us for the *"Best Possible Health."* **PLANTS** (grains, starches, beans, vegetables, and fruits) contain on average 5 to 10 percent fat, the ideal fat intake for the body.[4]

Plants have another benefit besides their low fat content: most are high in fiber. For the *"Best Possible Health,"* we need to eat at least 60 grams of fiber each day. The standard high-fat diet of animal foods provides fewer than 10 grams of fiber per day. Plant food contains a large amount of indigestible fiber that takes up twice as much space in the stomach for only half the calories of animal foods.[5]

High Fat Content In Animal Foods

There are *nine calories in each gram of fat*. Take a look at the fat content of some common animal foods: ground beef, 66 percent fat; bacon, 94 percent fat; whole milk, 48 percent fat; (2%) low-fat milk, 38 percent fat; cheddar cheese, 73 percent fat; eggs, 65 percent fat; T-bone steak, 82 percent fat; butter, 100 percent fat; and lard, 100 percent fat. Animal foods average more than 65 percent fat. Vegetable fats are just as bad. Don't delude yourself into thinking you've overcome the fat problem just because you're eating margarine instead of butter. Both are 100% fat. In butter you risk heart disease, and in margarine, cancer (see chapter 9). Be careful about products advertised as 80, 90, or 97 percent fat-free. Most labeling lists the percent fat by volume, not by the percent fat of calories as I will explain later. For example: Low fat (2%) milk is mostly water so this is a false percentage of nutrients. The true percentage of fat as a percentage of nutrients is 38%. See Appendix 1, USDA, Nutritive Value of Foods, 1988.

And what does your body do with all that fat? Remember, your body makes cholesterol from saturated fats and stores excess fat as fat.

Low Fat Content In Plant Foods

Now take a look at the fat content of some common plant foods: white potatoes, less than 1 percent fat; sweet potatoes, less than 1 percent fat; spaghetti (made from wheat), 5 percent fat; navy beans, 4 percent fat; brown rice, 4 percent fat; 100% whole wheat bread, about 13 percent fat; corn, 8 percent fat; and oatmeal, 12 percent fat. (Remember, however, to steer clear of olives, avocados, coconuts, chocolate, and most nuts and seeds except maybe as occasional treats.)

Are you eating the standard American diet? It consists of about 45 percent fat calories, 20 percent simple sugar calories, 20-25 percent protein calories, and 10-15 percent complex carbohydrate calories. It contains fewer than 10 grams of fiber per day, because there is absolutely no fiber in any animal food or simple sugar.[6]

Over The Millenia

Now look at *"The Miracle Diet"* Program, the same health plan that has been known for thousands of years. It contains approximately 10 percent fat, 10 percent protein, and 80 percent complex carbohydrate with 60 grams of indigestible fiber per day. You can, with few exceptions, eat all you can hold of plant foods, three meals per day, and snacks too, over a lifetime and never be overweight.

"The Miracle Diet" is easy to follow. You never have to count calories. Just eat starches instead of animal food for your entree or your main source of calories. Good choices include grains (wheat, oats, rice, corn, barley, rye), as well as potatoes and beans. Add vegetables and fruits to your starch-based diet, and soon you will learn to enjoy eating on the "Plantarian" program.[7]

The Other Effects of Fats

Obesity isn't the only problem related to too many dietary fats. Medical science has shown that fats cause a number of other problems, some of which are life-threatening.

When we eat a rich diet over a long period of time, the excess fat causes a great burden on our bodies. Eventually, our bodies fail to compensate for this burden, and disease and illness result.[8]

High Fat Levels Damage

1. Fats smother our tissues by cutting off their supply of oxygen.
2. Fats elevate our level of cholesterol and uric acid, causing atherosclerosis, gout and other chronic ailments.

3. Fats hinder our digestion of carbohydrates, causing adult diabetes.[9]

In excess, all fats (animal or vegetable, saturated or unsaturated) are bad for you. Ten percent or less fat calorie content in food is ideal. Fats also form a fatty film around the components of the blood, especially the red blood cells and platelets, causing them to stick together. After a fatty meal many small blood vessels become clogged, causing a shut down of up to 20 percent of the blood circulation and oxygen needed by our tissues for proper health. Eventually, the large blood vessels are diseased from lack of oxygen and restricted with fatty plaques, and this contributes to heart attacks, strokes, atherosclerosis, and many other diseases.[10]

Post Banquet Blahs Explained
Remember the last huge Thanksgiving dinner you ate and how listless and sleepy you got about an hour after that big meal. This condition is brought on by lack of oxygen to the brain and body tissues. This lack of oxygen caused by excessive fat in the bloodstream can also increase angina pains as the heart muscles cry out for more oxygen. Scientific studies have shown that patients suffering from heart disease can artificially bring on attacks of angina, or chest pain, by drinking a glass of cream or any vegetable oil.[11]

Body Cells Need Maximum Oxygen
Life is supported by the extraction of energy from food by a chemical process in the body that utilizes oxygen. Billions of cells in the body are fed oxygen by the lungs and the cardiovascular system. The body cannot live without oxygen.

Red blood cells are oxygenated in the lungs and they deliver their oxygen to the stationary tissue cells by going through the small narrow channels called capillaries. Without this process, nothing will work in our bodies. The red blood cell is shaped like a disc or round tire that is elastic and pliable. To deliver the oxygen into the body cells, the red cells squeeze single-file through the capillaries, the smallest blood vessels in the body. Because the capillaries are even smaller than the red blood cells themselves, they must expand to allow passage of the blood cells through them. Any clumping of red blood cells further restricts this passage.

When red cells transfer oxygen to the stationary cells, they also pick up waste carbon dioxide to be carried back to the lungs and exhaled. For this transfer or exchange to occur the red cells have to fit right up to the stationary cells, and that's why red cells must fit tightly as they pass through the capillaries. (Being elastic, the red cells can scrunch up enough to get through the tiny tubes one by one.)

Red Cell Clumping—Shortage of Oxygen

This whole process is very orderly, until we eat a big fatty meal. Then, the process is disrupted by the clumping, or sticking together, of the red cells. Fat gums up the circulation. It coats red cells and makes them stick together, a process that is called "rouleax formation."

Fats are not broken down by digestion into component parts, but are emulsified by bile acids into small droplets. Unlike amino acids and glucose, which are carried directly to the liver by the bloodstream, fats are absorbed by the lymphatic system, a slow-moving auxiliary circulation system to the blood system. The lymphatic stream bypasses the liver and dumps the fat into the blood stream at the level of the heart. From here fat is pumped by the heart all over the body. Therefore, if you eat an excessive amount of fat, you will get an excessive amount in your bloodstream.

As we eat more and more fat, the clumping of red cells continues to increase until there are masses of red cells that can't get through the capillaries. This process causes a serious reduction in the oxygen supply to the body tissues. Some researchers say up to a 30 percent shutdown in our oxygen transfer takes place. Our entire body is heavily burdened by this shortage of oxygen.[12]

Seven

Milk:
DOES it do a body good?

Dr. Russell Bunai, a noted Washington D.C. pediatrician was asked what single dietary change would benefit America the most. His answer may stun you. . . . He said, *"Eliminate dairy products."*[1] Bunai is one of a rapidly growing corps of physicians, nutritionists and researchers who have begun to see that cow's milk is a food we should do without.

Let's examine the soundness of these doctor's views by first examining some "extras" that come along with today's milk.

The Modern Dairy Farm—
America's Pharmaceutical Dumping Ground

A 1990 article in the Washington Post asked, "How safe is the milk we drink?" It reported on Congressional hearings in which Food and Drug Administration officials reported testing 70 retail milk samples in 14 cities. Fifty-one percent were contaminated with antibiotics and sulfa drugs.

Post columnist Coleman McCarthy comments, "The bad news is that the milk industry can't say no to drugs. In the pharmaceutical barnyard, commercial cows are bred for profits and then chemicalized to maximize production at minimum cost."

Unfortunately, this was not just an isolated incident.

- A March 1988 survey by the Food and Drug Administration revealed that 36 out of 49 samples of milk collected from 10 cities were contaminated with sulfamethazine, a drug that prevents bacterial growth and that has never been legally approved for use in lactating dairy cows.

- Surveys by independent researchers found that more than 60 percent of retail milk samples contained measurable levels of other antimicrobials including sulfonamides, tetracycline, streptomycin, and chloramphenicol. . . .

  The Wall Street Journal collected 50 samples from 10 cities around the country [And] 38 percent were contaminated with low levels of sulfonamides. streptomycin, penicillin, or erythromycin . . .

  In the wake of the survey results reported in the Wall Street Journal, the FDA has tested 70 samples of milk from 14 cities and 36 (over 50 percent) of the samples contained drug residues.

- 85 of 120 or 71% of the samples from milk transport tanker trucks and off retail shelves in six New England states were contaminated with sulfamethazine or other sulfonamide residues.

- 40 of 64 or 63% of retail milk samples from three Northeastern states were contaminated, mostly with tetracyclines and sulfonamides.

- 150 of 174 or 86% of retail milk samples from 16 states and 29 of 40 or 73% of retail Canadian samples were contaminated mostly with tetracycline and sulfonamides.[2]

Of course, some drugs are more harmful than others, and some people are more sensitive to certain drugs than others, but consider chloramphenicol. This drug "is banned from ever being used in food-producing animals," but it "has been detected in milk, according to published reports by independent researchers, and was also recently found on 5 of 78 Colorado dairy farms." Chloramphenicol is "a powerful antibiotic" and is "associated with aplastic anemia, an irreversible and potentially fatal bone-marrow disease."[3]

A March 28, 1994 *Newsweek* article criticized the dairy industry for its overuse of chemicals. It stated, "For sheer over-prescription, no doctor can touch the American farmer. Farm animals receive 30 times more antibiotics than people do."

Nursing—
Great for Babies, but Everyone Should Quit Sometime

Washington Post columnist, Coleman McCarthy, also wrote in his 1988 investigation, "While cows are being raised as if they were junkies, the public is sedated by the self-serving National Dairy Council that for seventy-five years has been hyping milk as nature's most perfect food. If that's the case, why aren't cows drinking it? After weaning, nature guides them (cows) to water. Humans are the sole species that consume milk—and not even its own kind—past infancy." He correctly asks, "What nutritional wisdom do we have that has been denied all the rest of nature?"[4]

It seems that whole cow's milk is, indeed, a "perfect food," but only if you are a baby cow. Milk is high in fat (nearly 50 percent fat calories) and loaded with cholesterol. Milk contains absolutely no fiber and is low in carbohydrates. When you look at the nutrient make-up of milk, it is so similar to animal flesh that it might be referred to as "liquid meat."

Milk, Diabetes and Multiple Sclerosis

Juvenile diabetes has been linked to the consumption of cow's milk by individuals who have a susceptibility to the disease. Children who are not exposed to cow's milk early in life have a dramatically lower risk. (see Chapter 10 on diabetes)

In John Robbin's Book *Diet for a New America,* he states, "Children who are fed cow's milk formulas grow up into adults with a higher susceptiblity to Multiple Sclerosis."

Around the world the incidence of MS and the consumption of dairy products seems to be directly proportional.

Allergies—NOT Just from Pollen and Dust

Researchers have found that dairy products are the leading cause of food allergies.[5] They contain more than twenty-five different proteins that induce allergic reactions in humans.[6]

Scientists admit that after the age of four years, most people naturally lose the ability to digest the carbohydrate in milk known as lactose, because they no longer synthesize the digestive enzyme lactase, which lines the small intestine. This is known medically as lactose intolerance, and causes diarrhea, gas, and stomach cramps when dairy products are consumed. Scientists say that in adult Asians and blacks worldwide there is as much as a 90 percent rate of intolerance to animal milk products. There is also as much as a 60 percent rate of intolerance among Mexicans and Eskimos, and about 20 percent intolerance rate among the white population of the world.[7]

Milk and Your Heart

According to the U.S. Department of Agriculture, milk products in general contain about 60 percent saturated fat and even many of the so-called "low-fat" milk products have a relatively high fat calorie content. (see Appendix I).

Cholesterol in the diet causes heart-artery disease, heart attacks and strokes. The saturated fat in milk is converted by the human liver into cholesterol which may be even more damaging to the blood vessels than cholesterol that is ingested directly. Dr. Neal D. Barnard says, "As far as cholesterol is concerned, the bottom line is that saturated fats are the worst cholesterol-makers."[8]

The Calcium Myth

With all these problems, why do we continue to buy milk? There are two highly publicized "reasons." The first and foremost is calcium, and the second is Vitamin-D.

We are barraged daily with advertising telling us that for healthy bones and teeth we "must" get our calcium from milk products. Think about this one for a minute—*Where do cows get the calcium they eat?* They get it from plants, and so should we! Plants happen to contain just the right amount of calcium for the ideal health of both humans and cows.

Billions of people in Asia and Africa rarely drink milk, yet they have strong bones and sturdy teeth. As an added bonus, these nonconsumers of milk products do not suffer the degenerative diseases that are common in the affluent, milk-consuming nations of North America and Europe.

Women in the African Bantu society are excellent examples. They use no milk products but consume from 250 to 400 mg. of calcium per day from plant sources. *That's only 25% of the current*

USDA Recommended Daily Allowance! They commonly have ten babies during their lifetime, and breast feed each child for nearly a year. Despite all of this calcium drain and relatively low calcium intake, osteoporosis is still basically unknown among native Bantu women. However, if these same women move to affluent animal-eating societies and begin eating rich foods, osteoporosis and diseases of the teeth become common among them. They have no genetic guarantees.[9]

Noted author and researcher, Dr. John McDougall, says, "The calcium present in the diet has little effect on the quality of calcium that is eventually taken into the body. The intestine absorbs, from the foods consumed, sufficient calcium to meet the needs of the body. On low-calcium diets the efficiency of absorption is increased, and on high-calcium diets less absorption occurs. Unprocessed vegetable foods contain sufficient calcium to meet the needs of adults and growing children. In fact, calcium deficiency caused by an insufficient amount of calcium in the diet is not known to occur in humans, even though most people in the world don't drink milk after weaning because of custom, lactose intolerance, or unavailability. Consider this the next time you hear the dairy industry's favorite advertising pitch about the necessity of drinking milk to meet calcium needs."

The final irony is that much calcium is leached from our bones because of the high animal protein that comes along with milk. A high protein diet causes leaching of calcium from the bones that is then lost by being excreted in the urine. (see Chapter 8 on Osteoporosis)

What About the Vitamin D Argument?

According to scientists, vitamin D is really not a vitamin, because the body can and does under most circumstances make, or synthesize, all that it needs. Vitamin D is a hormone synthesized by the action of sunlight on plant sterols found in the skin. Our body levels of vitamin D are only slightly affected by dietary sources, such as milk fortified with vitamin D and vitamin supplements. The disease of rickets is a disorder characterized by painful and deformed bones. This disease is common in places where there is a limited exposure to sunlight. Because vitamin D is fat-soluble, this hormone can be stored in body fat for long periods of time, and intermittent exposure to sunlight is adequate. There are hundreds of scientific references on the subject of milk consumption and health problems in the Western world's rich-food society. I have quoted from only a few of them.[10]

Who's Messing with your Mind?

Finally, consider why it is that we as a culture use dairy products to the extent we do. Is there a financial interest at work that want's us to consume milk regardless of its negative health consequences?

In *Diet for A New America,* John Robbins describes the aggressiveness with which the Dairy Council (the dairy industry's public relations and advertising arm) has penetrated schools with the one-sided message that milk is wholesome, while ignoring that many independent nutritionists' report the serious diseases and allergies that are brought on by high-cholesterol, high-fat and high-protein dairy products.

All the items that are made from cow's milk—cheese, butter, cottage cheese, yogurt, buttermilk, skim milk, ice cream, whey (a cheese production waste-product that is "recycled" into our food and used in a host of other products), and cow's milk-based baby formulas—are the life's blood of a multi-billion dollar industry.

The use of dairy products is on a downward trend therefore, the dairy industry has recently launched a $50-million-dollar "milk mustache" advertising campaign to make sure America keeps buying one of nature's most *imperfect* foods for humans.

The psychology behind their pitch is brilliant. Dr. Steven Locke, Instructor in Psychiatry and Director of the Psycho-immunology Research Project at Harvard Medical School said in a 1988 New York Times interview, "We are moved from mother's milk to cow's milk very early in life, so that the taste of cow's milk is associated with being held next to mother's breast. Milk has a bigger-than-life image because it's linked to mothering in ways that only Madison Avenue (the advertising industry) could appreciate."

Eight

Osteoporosis:
Our Love Affair With Meat, Eggs, and Milk

It's been reported that 55% of all women, in America, 50 years of age and older suffer from some form of osteoporosis. Osteoporosis is perhaps the most misunderstood and among the most serious medical problems women are likely to face. It has nothing to do with cholesterol or fat. And it's not prevented by drinking plenty of milk. Its sinister presence lies in the realm of protein metabolism—and its prevention lies in a plant-centered diet.

Dr. Harrison's 1977 edition of *Principles of Internal Medicine* contains a chapter on osteoporosis. It states, "Another factor which some have implicated in bone loss is the possibility that excessive acid intake, particularly in the form of high-protein diets, results in "dissolution" of bone in an attempt to buffer the extra acid."[1]

We now know that Harrison's succinctly stated theory is true; it's been documented by 20 years of scientific medical evidence.[2]

Too Much Protein

Osteoporosis is the term used to describe a variety of diseases characterized by a reduction in the mass of bone to a level below that required for adequate mechanical support of the body.

However, the **common cause** of this devastating disease is too much protein in the diet (over 15%) and a sedentary lifestyle. Most Americans consume over 20% protein daily.

Excessive amounts of proteins (especially from animal foods) cause changes in kidney activity, resulting in large losses of calcium from the body.

Studies have shown that protein levels commonly consumed by Americans will cause more calcium to be lost from the body than can be absorbed from the gut, even when the person is consuming very high levels of calcium. Phosphates from sodas (such as cola drinks) and caffeine also cause calcium losses.

Nursing babies only get 5% protein in mother's milk yet the greatest need of protein is in the first year after birth. This demonstrates that humans need a relatively small amount of protein. We have been misled by the Dairy and Beef Lobbies, and many well intentioned but misinformed healthcare providers.

The common form of osteoporosis is caused by the **excessive loss of calcium**. It is the result of long-standing ingestion of excess animal protein and lack of exercise.[3] Let me explain. Eating too much protein with its high amino acid content will load the body excessively with acids. In order to maintain a critical level of acid-alkaline balance for thousands of orderly functions, the body must neutralize this excess acid and does so by buffering (neutralizing) it with calcium robbed from the bones. In this process, calcium is taken out of the bones and excreted in the urine. It is a disease of calcium loss. It is **NOT** a calcium deficiency. As one expert states, "There is no difference in the calcium intake of (the) osteoporotic compared with control subjects of similar age and sex."[4]

A plant-centered diet, with its high-complex carbohydrate content, its high fiber content, its minerals, including calcium and vitamins and especially its *low but essential protein content is* necessary for the body and *is the preventive diet* against the tragedy of osteoporosis.

Need for Physical Activity

Another factor in the prevention of osteoporosis is exercise. This is best illustrated by what happens to bedridden people. They lose calcium in their bones very rapidly and are prone to bone fractures. However, the more the bones in the arm, leg, or back are used, the stronger they become because activity helps deposit calcium into the bones.

In our society there are other obvious conditions that make an individual more susceptible to osteoporosis. The alcoholics, who get a large portion of calories from alcohol and fail to get proper nourishment can become osteoporotic. Smokers, whose appetites are diminished and who eat poorly, also are susceptible. Drinking three cups of coffee containing caffeine triples calcium loss to the urine for the next several hours.

The Best Prevention

While this disease is widespread in our affluent Western society osteoporosis is virtually nonexistent in billions of people in Africa and Asia where animal products are rarely eaten and milk products are virtually unknown. For example, the Chinese eat mainly rice, potatoes, beans, corn, wheat, barley, oats, fruit and vegetables. Their babies are breast fed and then weaned. The bones and teeth of both children and adults are strong and healthy.

The dairy industry has scared most women into using milk products indicating they will surely suffer from osteoporosis if they don't get their calcium from milk. Ironically, the exact opposite is true! Milk products are high in protein and high protein intake is the common cause of osteoporosis. It only stands to reason, if you take in high amounts of protein your body will leach the calcium from your bones and cause osteoporosis.

The average American eats from two to five times as much protein as he or she needs. The daily protein intake of Americans is 90-120 grams and represents about 25% of total calories consumed. The ideal protein intake is 20-40 grams per day, representing about 10% of total calories. The World Health Organization recommends 37 grams of protein per day and good scientific data shows that 20 grams will maintain positive nitrogen balance—a measure of adequate protein.[5]

We need to reduce our intake of protein and become "Plantarian." Knowing the cause of osteoporosis enables us to design a lifelong program of prevention centered on the truths taught in *"The Miracle Diet"* food plan.

As has been previously stated, cows and other animals get their calcium from the plants they eat and humans should get their calcium from plants, too.

Nine

Cancer Prevention— the Best Cure

The American Cancer Society and medical complex seem to be selling "hope" when it comes to cancer. This subject is not a pleasant one but for your future protection from needless pain and suffering you should carefully read and digest this chapter on cancer. It may save your life!

Cancer is the number two killer (behind heart-artery diseases) and accounts for nearly 24 percent of deaths each year. In 1995 about 547,000 Americans will die of cancer—nearly 1,500 people a day. One out of every five deaths in the US is from cancer. The National Cancer Institute estimates $35 billion for direct medical treatment costs and overall costs at $104 billion for just one year.[1]

Over the past decade John A. McDougall, M.D., researcher and writer, has been associating the type of food we eat with the many degenerative diseases we suffer from in America and other affluent countries. His review of scientific literature of this century has convinced him and many others that plant food promotes health, and that animal foods and added fats promote disease and death.

In his 1985 book, *McDougall's Medicine: A Challenging Second Opinion*, Dr. McDougall covers the subject of cancer in great detail. Everyone should read this important well-documented scientific information. In 1989, Dr. McDougall made a series of audio tapes, one of which candidly covers the subject of cancer. Much of the information in this chapter is based on his writings and tapes.

The Physiology of Common Cancers

When the human body functions properly, cells divide whenever a neighboring cell dies, thus maintaining a healthy balance. Cancer cells, however, do not follow the rules of cell division. Cancer begins with a single cell which divides in approximately one hundred days to make two cancer cells. And this doubling process goes on every one hundred days. A year later, a mass of twelve cancer cells has developed in, for example, a woman's breast or a man's prostate gland. There is no way to detect this tumor because it is microscopic.

The doubling continues so that after six years a mass of one million cells has developed, only one millimeter in size; about the size of a pinhead. This mass is still not detectable by any present method. It is still too small. Research indicates that if cancer has been in the body for six years, there is a 90 percent chance that it has been carried by the bloodstream to other locations, and that the doubling rate has begun again somewhere else.

Mammography cannot usually detect a breast mass until it has been in the breast for about eight years. After mathematically doubling for ten years, cancer of the breast contains one billion cells. At that time the lump is detectable by palpation, and is usually discovered by the patient herself.

Long-term medical studies on the results of breast cancer treatment have proved very disappointing. In the past fifty-five years, the death rate from breast cancer, prostate cancer, colon cancer, and other organ cancers has not decreased at all.

Experts say it is not the tumor in the breast that kills, but the cancer that has spread to other parts of the body (the bones, brain, liver, or lungs) all from a single cell that has metastasized from the breast. Finally, cancer is not toxic in and of itself, but it destroys a vital organ of the body by replacing healthy tissue with cancer cells.[2]

The Causes and the Cures

With disappointing cure rates for cancer, prevention is the only intelligent alternative. And the best method of prevention is *"The Miracle Diet"* program.

People believe that many things contribute to cancer: preservatives in foods, contamination, radiation, and chemicals in the soil, to name a few. There are elements of truth in all of these things, but the major causes of cancer are the major things in our lives. What could be more "major" than the one to five pounds of food we eat each day? That is what provides the greatest contact between our bodies and our environment. In 1988, U.S. Surgeon General C. Everett Koop announced that what we eat **DOES** cause cancer.

The air we breathe and the water we drink have a significant impact on our health, but *food* is by far the most important component of our environment, and the most controllable. The type of food we eat has the most direct impact on our health.

Macro-nutrients (carbohydrates, protein and fat), have the greatest influence on the cause of most common cancers. Vitamins and minerals are micro-nutrients that contribute to our health, however, it's the percentage of macro-nutrients and fiber that are by far the major components of our diet. They have the greatest bearing on whether we enjoy good health or suffer from sickness and unnecessary disease.

You've heard the old adage, "You are what you eat." This literally is true. The food we eat ends up as part of every cell of the body. The fat component of our diet is the prime suspect in most common cancers in America.

Cancers in Men and Women

A study group for the National Academy of Science recently reviewed a large body of evidence that supported the claim made by investigators worldwide that 60 percent of female cancers and 40 percent of cancers found in men are related to diet.[3]

Women suffer from breast cancer, colon cancer, ovarian cancer, and body of the uterus cancer. These are associated with high fat in the diet which affects the hormonal balance. Men suffer from prostate cancer and colon cancer, and both are associated with a high fat intake. Both sexes are subject to pancreatic cancer which is mostly associated with high fat intake. Lymphomas have been associated with excess dairy protein which stimulates the immune system to a point where it breaks down.

Researchers continue to point to our diet as the major cause of breast cancer in women. In 1990, 150,000 American women were diagnosed with breast cancer. In 1995 the estimated number has dramatically increased to 182,000.[4] As we eat more and more fast foods containing large amounts of animal products and as we add more and more vegetable fat to our diets, we accelerate the rate of breast cancer. This surely must be true in the case of all other diet-related cancers, such as cancer of the ovary, uterus, colon, pancreas, prostate, as well as lymphomas.

Leukemia and Lung Cancer

Some experts suspect that leukemia may, in some cases, be caused by a bovine leukemia virus that is transmitted from cows to humans through milk. There is still much to investigate, but the highest rates of leukemia are in the countries that consume the most dairy products.

Is it possible that lung cancer could have a connection to diet? Smoking is of course a major cause, but other factors may be involved, too. Research has shown smokers with high cholesterol levels have a seven times greater cancer rate as those with low cholesterol levels who smoke the same amount of cigarettes.

Immunize Yourself Against Cancer

Researchers have reported vitamin A intake, especially the vegetable beta carotene type of vitamin A, is important. Smokers who consume very few plant foods have eight times as many lung cancers as those who consume a high amount of vegetables, and smoke the same amount. If you take in a noxious substance, your body can better fight it off if you are in good health.[5]

In mid-1990, following a seven-year study, University of Arizona immunologist, Ronald Watson, and his team of researchers concluded that beta carotene, an antioxidant found in many vegetables, boosts the immune system's attack on cancer cells. The UA team said that's because beta carotene stirs up natural killer cells, immune-system cells that hunt for rampaging cancer cells before they can settle down and become a tumor. The compound dramatically increases the number of immune-system cells and spurs the production of proteins that kill cancer. This means that the antioxidant, beta carotene, may help prevent some types of cancer, although it probably won't be of much use against already established tumors.

The scientists documented interesting changes in immune-system cells exposed to beta carotene, which is used by the body to make vitamin A. The UA researchers showed in laboratory mice and test tubes that beta carotene makes killer cells much more efficient at dispatching cancer cells. They say there is much more work to be done on human cancer prevention and beta carotene, but in the meantime we should all eat our vegetables.[6]

Some societies consume low-fat diets and smoke heavily, and have relatively low rates of lung cancer. Japan and Turkey are two good examples. Both have low rates of lung cancer compared to the United States. Japan and Turkey both follow a traditional, mostly plant-based diet.[7]

Colon Cancer

One in twenty people in America will suffer from colon cancer. This disease has been linked to a diet high in fat. It only makes sense to suspect that the one to five pounds of food we run through our colon each day could be the culprit.

As previously stated, world-famous researcher Dr. Denis Burkitt has taught for many years that it is the lack of fiber in our diet that is implicated in the cause of colon cancer and many other diseases of the intestinal tract.[8] Animal food must be the culprit in the case of fiber, because there is absolutely NO fiber in any flesh or animal by-product. The animal food we eat is devoid of fiber, and as our main intake of calories naturally causes small concentrated stools in our bowel. We call this constipation. This small stool lies in our bowel for up to 72 hours or more, during which time concentrated substances and carcinogens in the stool remnant irritate and enhance the chance for developing colon cancer. Most people think that as long as we have one bowel movement each day, no matter the amount or concentration, there is no problem. When there is sufficient fiber in the diet, you will generally have one or more large, loose, non-concentrated bowel movements each day. It is virtually impossible to be constipated when you eat plants as your main source of calories. The high fiber we get in plant foods quickly dilute and flush away the many carcinogens and cancer-causing materials before they can damage the colon walls.[9]

The second most deadly cancerous disease in America is that of the colon and rectum. It is rampant because of two dietary factors: inadequate fiber and excess fat. The relationship between dietary fat and death from colon cancer is shown in the following graph.

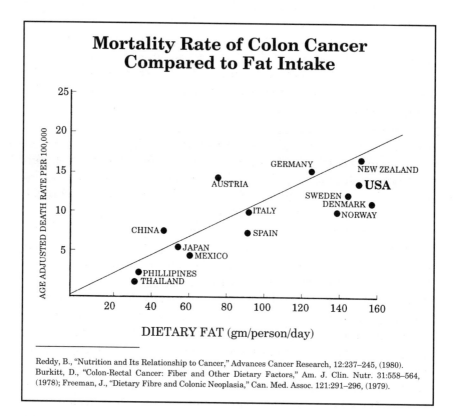

Mortality Rate of Colon Cancer Compared to Fat Intake

Reddy, B., "Nutrition and Its Relationship to Cancer," Advances Cancer Research, 12:237–245, (1980). Burkitt, D., "Colon-Rectal Cancer: Fiber and Other Dietary Factors," Am. J. Clin. Nutr. 31:558–564, (1978); Freeman, J., "Dietary Fibre and Colonic Neoplasia," Can. Med. Assoc. 121:291–296, (1979).

Countries with a high-fiber, plant-centered diet (lots of grain, rice, corn, beans, and potatoes) have the lowest death rates from colon cancer.[10] Numerous studies confirm the long standing declaration of Dr. Denis Burkitt that low fiber in food is the offender.[11] Recent studies suggest that a high-fat diet and low-fiber diet allow carcinogens to remain in contact longer with the bowel wall. Fecal bile acids and fecal cholesterol have been incriminated as co-carcinogens in these studies.

Do You Want to be Shot or Hung?

Research scientists have fed high-fat diets to animals and produced high rates of cancer. Interestingly, the very best way to produce cancer faster, with more tumors, is to feed the animals high amounts of *vegetable fat.*[12] As cited earlier, vegetable fats like shortening and cooking oils are rather new in our society. As their use has dramatically increased, the rate of breast cancer has jumped by 100 percent in the last 30 years.[13] According to the National Cancer Institute, the U.S. incidence rate increased 32 percent in only five years between 1982 and 1987.[14]

Other researchers have noted that wherever people ate high amounts of cholesterol and had high rates of heart disease, they also had high rates of colon cancer. Animal experiments have shown the same relationship. The more cholesterol that is fed to animals, the more tumors are produced and the faster the animals died of cancer. Cholesterol and saturated fats cause heart disease whereas all fats, especially vegetable fats, contribute to major cancers in this country. If you substitute vegetable fat for animal fat you essentially may be making a choice between risking heart disease or cancer. It's like choosing to be either shot or hung. Neither alternative is attractive.

Other research concludes that animal protein causes colon cancer because protein gets converted to cancer-causing substances which end up in the colon.

Still other researchers have found that if they feed cabbage, cauliflower, broccoli and other cruciferous vegetables to animals that are simultaneously being injected with cancer-causing chemicals, it is difficult to cause colon cancer in these animals. The vegetables in the cabbage family contain cancer inhibiting compounds.[15] Scientists now refer to these immune-system enhancing substances as phytochemicals. They are being widely studied and isolated to be used as food supplements. Phytochemicals are only found in plant foods and seem to be much more potent in their natural form. This proves the wisdom of *"The Miracle Diet."*

Women and Colon Cancer

The largest study of Western world diets and colon cancer was conducted over a six-year period and involved 88,751 women ranging in age from 34 to 59. It found that the more red meat and animal fat consumed, the more likely the development of this common and deadly cancer. (December 12, 1990, *New England Journal of Medicine*).

Researchers said the study offered strong evidence that diet is an important factor in determining who gets colon cancer. They reported that those eating animal fat products every day were more than twice as likely to develop colon cancer as those who ate animal fat products once a month.[16]

Breast Cancer—Danger Ahead!

In 1960, thirty-five years ago, one in twenty American women developed breast cancer. By 1990 one in ten women developed breast cancer.[17] By 1993 these statistics had increased shockingly to one in eight women. This clearly points out that when women eat nearly 50% fat calories each day the risk of developing deadly breast cancer greatly increases. There is a straight-line correlation between the amount of animal food and fat we eat and deaths from breast cancer (Figure 1).

You find high rates of breast cancer in the same affluent countries where colon cancer and heart disease are common. People in these countries consume large amounts of dairy products, eggs, and animals, just as you would expect. The wealthy countries of United Kingdom, the Netherlands, Australia, Canada, the United States, and Sweden experience high rates of breast cancer. Poor countries like Columbia, Ceylon (Sri Lanka) and Thailand have low rates of breast cancer—about one-sixth that of The U.S.[18] Breast cancer is now one of the fastest growing diseases among Japanese women, with incidence up 58 percent in only 10 years between 1975 and 1985. [19] It has increased at about the same rate as the Japanese have added more fat to their diet since the end of World War II. Looking at the dietary changes of Japanese women who moved to Hawaii following the war makes a strong argument for the importance of diet to breast cancer.

While they continued to eat their basic traditional diet of rice and vegetables, Japanese women who moved to Hawaii after the war also ate more fat than they had in Japan. Just the small increase in dietary fats caused the Japanese women in Hawaii to have twice the incidence of breast cancer compared to women in Japan. Researchers found that by increasing fat intake only slightly above 10 percent, a woman increases her breast cancer risk.

In 1974, researchers looked at Japanese women living in California who were completely Americanized. The incidence of breast cancer among the Japanese-American women living in the San Francisco Bay Area of California was exactly the same as it was for the Caucasian women in that same area. Their genes had not changed, but the women had changed their diet.

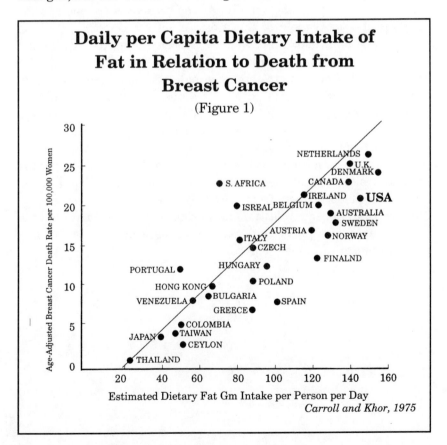

Daily per Capita Dietary Intake of Fat in Relation to Death from Breast Cancer

(Figure 1)

Carroll and Khor, 1975

Since the end of World War II, fast food restaurants have come to Japan, and the Japanese have begun to Westernize their diet. They also started to get heart disease and gall bladder disease, virtually unknown before the war.

In Japan researchers studied women who became wealthy and started eating meat at least seven times a week and compared them to women living in small villages who ate the traditional Japanese diet of rice and vegetables and a little fish. What researchers found was amazing but not unexpected: the difference in the rate of breast cancer in these two groups of women was 850 percent![20]

Prostate Cancer is Deadly

Men are not exempt from a hormonal type of cancer. Cancer of the prostate is increasing rapidly. At the present time, one in nine men will develop cancer of the prostate. Of all cancers, only lung cancer kills more men than prostate cancer. Again, as with breast cancer, prostate cancer is linked to hormones, obesity and a high-fat diet. In this instance, testosterone, a male hormone is incriminated. Men, who consume more fat, are more prone to develop prostate cancer.[21] (See Figure 2 on next page.) A plant-centered diet reduces blood testosterone levels.[22] Scientists have for years been interested in members of the Seventh-day Adventist Church because of its plant-centered tradition. Adventist men have only one-third the prostate cancer risk of other men. The non-obese male has a lower death rate than the obese from prostate cancer.[23]

Prostate cancer is relatively unknown in populations around the world that eat a plant-centered diet. Plantarians have far less prostate cancer than meat-eaters.

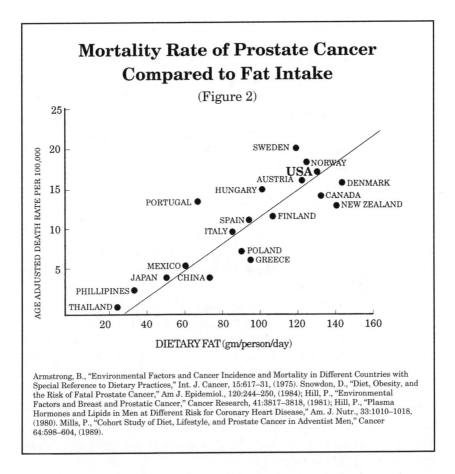

**Mortality Rate of Prostate Cancer
Compared to Fat Intake**
(Figure 2)

Armstrong, B., "Environmental Factors and Cancer Incidence and Mortality in Different Countries with Special Reference to Dietary Practices," Int. J. Cancer, 15:617–31, (1975). Snowdon, D., "Diet, Obesity, and the Risk of Fatal Prostate Cancer," Am J. Epidemiol., 120:244–250, (1984); Hill, P., "Environmental Factors and Breast and Prostatic Cancer," Cancer Research, 41:3817–3818, (1981); Hill, P., "Plasma Hormones and Lipids in Men at Different Risk for Coronary Heart Disease," Am. J. Nutr., 33:1010–1018, (1980). Mills, P., "Cohort Study of Diet, Lifestyle, and Prostate Cancer in Adventist Men," Cancer 64:598–604, (1989).

Diet and Hormones

Elevated estrogen levels increase a woman's risk of breast cancer, and elevated levels of sex hormones in men increase the risk of cancer of the prostate gland. [24] Some researchers say stored cholesterol in the body also creates deterioration of the prostate gland by forming cholesterol crystals in the gland.[25]

With too much estrogen, women's breasts become lumpy and tender; called fibrocystic breast disease, more than one-half of all American women have it. Often the cells in the breast break down, and cancer of the breast results. The over-stimulation of the uterus by excessive estrogen causes 30 percent of women in America to lose their uterus by post-menopausal time.[26]

The cause? Most researchers agree it is too much fat in the diet!

Animal studies done years ago show that when animals are fed high-fat diets, cancers grow faster. If animals are fed low-fat, no-cholesterol diets, cancer growth is retarded and animals live longer. According to medical literature, other studies show that obese women with high cholesterol levels have triple the death rate of women who are thin and who have low cholesterol.

Cancer is Caused by What We Eat

Many of these facts have been in the scientific literature for a long time but have not received enough attention. In 1977, the Senate Select Committee on Nutrition was the first large group to come out and tell us that the American diet was causally related to breast and colon cancer.

In 1979, the National Cancer Institute said the way to reduce your chances of cancer was to eat a low-fat, high-fiber diet.

Then in 1982, the National Academy of Science stated that the major cancers in men and women are caused by what we eat: the high-fat, low-fiber, high-cholesterol diet.

The American Cancer Society in 1984 spoke out and said, "If you want to reduce your risk of cancer you need to cut your intake of meat and dairy products, and you should increase your intake of grains, vegetables, and fruits, as well as decrease your fat intake from forty percent to thirty percent."[27]

This is at least recognizing the problem, but who really knows the exact percentage of fat in the food we eat? Maybe not one in a million. Do you know how much fat, protein, or carbohydrate is in the different foods you eat each meal or in between meals? It's easy if you follow *"The Miracle Diet"* program. (See Appendix 1).. You will automatically be getting between 5 and 10 percent fat if you eat basically plant foods. This gives you the maximum protection from all food-related cancers and many other diseases that are nearly 100 percent preventable.[28]

Prevention The Best Cure

In his 1990 book, *The Power of Your Plate,* Neal D. Barnard, M.D., emphasized that cancer prevention is all important. "From my own prospective, an optimal diet for cancer prevention means cutting back or eliminating meats and dairy products, which are devoid of fiber and frequently much too high in fat and protein. It means avoiding fried foods and added oils. And it means having generous amounts of whole grains, legumes, and vegetables. Any shift toward this optimal diet is a shift toward health," he said.

Dr. Barnard quotes from other noted scientific medical leaders and researchers. Dr. Oliver Alabaster, M.D., director of the Institute for Disease Prevention at George Washington University Medical Center says, "At least 70 percent of cancer is thought to be preventable. Changing dietary habits requires people to be willing to take steps now to reduce their risk of something years ahead." Dr. Alabaster asks fellow physicians to be agents of information: "It requires physicians to realize that they have a responsibility to try to prevent disease as well as to treat it, something which is usually under-emphasized in medical education."

Preventive Measures—The Way of the Future

Dr. Alabaster also said, "Preventive measures are really the way of the future. They have also been the way of the past. A hundred years ago, half the population was dead before the age of forty, mainly because of infection. Now that number is down to three percent, entirely due to preventive measures: better sanitation, better hygiene, vaccinations, and to a very small extent, direct therapy. This is a dramatic change produced by preventive measures. The three major killer diseases that now account for premature mortality are cancer, heart disease and stroke. They account for four out of five deaths. Yet these three diseases are largely untreatable and almost entirely preventable if we make the right decisions. So the three major killer diseases which will otherwise be with us well into the next century could be abolished if we take the right steps."

Meat is a Relatively New Phenomenon

"Our modern diet is really an anathema to our whole historical evolution," Alabaster said. "Why should we expect our bodies to react well to it? In the evolutionary time-scale meat is a relatively new phenomenon. It used to be fruit, nuts, cereal, and vegetation were really the basis of the human diet over the millennia. The good news is that we now realize that we can, to a great degree, control our risks of cancer and other diseases through decisions we make ourselves. I hope we will take advantage of it." [29]

Cancer May Be 90% Preventable

Dr. Oliver Alabaster wrote in his book *The Power of Prevention* that, environmental factors such as diet and smoking are now thought to cause as much as 90 percent of all human cancer in the United States, which means that cancer is potentially a *preventable disease.*

Statistics show that smoking causes 30 percent of all deaths; therefore the way we eat is largely responsible for 60 percent of all deaths in the United States. Those statistics bear an important message: *cancer is preventable.* Dr. Alabaster wrote further,

The inability of a smoker to quit is as understandable as the inability of a compulsive eater to close a box of Swiss chocolate. Yet these forms of neurotic compulsion are not the reason we fail to make sensible adjustments in our diet. What we have always lacked is *informed guidance.* This situation has now changed. You can lessen your risk of cancer by planned changes in your diet . . . A cancer prevention diet should become the normal diet for everyone . . . We need not take into consideration every known food chemical and its possible interaction with other chemicals . . . Every day there are women who endure the physical and psychological mutilation of a radical mastectomy (breast removal) for a cancer that may have been caused by excessive fat in the diet.[29] (emphasis added)

Dr. Barnard's steps to cancer prevention are: Do not use tobacco in any form. Limit fat intake to 10 percent of total calories including all types of fats and oils. Increase fiber to 40-60 grams daily by including more whole grains, beans, and vegetables in the diet.

Minimize or, preferably, eliminate foods from animal sources. Increase intake of dark green, orange and yellow vegetables. Especially, make cruciferous vegetables, such as broccoli, brussels sprouts, cabbage, and cauliflower a regular part of your diet. Maintain your weight at or near ideal weight. Avoid exposure to excessive sunlight or unnecessary x-rays.[29]

THE "New Four Food Groups," 1991

The Physicians Committee For Responsible Medicine, a national organization headquartered in Washington, D.C., has launched a massive educational program to teach school children and adults that eating mostly plant foods with virtually no added fats creates optimum health. The Committee has available full-color, 22" X 17" posters depicting The **"New Four Food Groups"** which replaces the old, outdated 1956 Four Basic Food Groups. Many other educational materials are available. One of the materials is The Gold Plan, a unique nutritional education program for hospitals, schools, universities, businesses, and other institutions. This Plan is designed to meet consumer demands for healthful and delicious food, and encourages people to choose healthful cafeteria meals. All of this material will make it easier to improve eating habits. For information call (202) 686-2210 or write: Physicians Committee For Responsible Medicine, P.O. Box 6322, Washington, D.C. 20016, Neal D. Barnard, M.D., President.[30]

Personal Habits Get in Our Way

Scientists who themselves eat meat sometimes have a difficult time being objective about the potential negative effects of meat on human health. This situation can produce "scientific conclusions" that are slanted in the wrong direction. Men of science are human, too. However, enough scientific literature does exist that shows clearly the relationship between high fat intake and many common cancers. When we are involved in eating foods that cause disease, it is hard to accept those foods as the cause of a problem.[31]

People defend their personal habits. Are we rationalizing our current habit of eating rich animal foods and killing ourselves in the process?

For More Information

For more detailed information on major degenerative diseases and how to avoid and even cure them, John A. McDougall, M.D. has published four informative and well-written books:

- *"The McDougall Plan,"* by John A. McDougall, M.D. and Mary McDougall, New Century Publishers, 1983.
- *"McDougall's Medicine: A Challenging Second Opinion,"* by John A. McDougall, M.D., New Century Publishers, 1985.
- *"The McDougall Program: Twelve Days to Dynamic Health,"* by John A. McDougall, M.D., National Books Publisher, 1990.
- *"The McDougall Program for Maximum Weight Loss,"* by John A. McDougall, M.D., Plume Publishing, 1995.

Audio and video tapes are also available from the McDougalls, P. O. Box 14039, Santa Rosa, California 95402, or call (707) 576-1654.

A twelve-day live-in health program is conducted by Dr. McDougall at St. Helena's Health Center, Deer Park, California 94576. Call (800) 358-9195 (outside California) or (800) 862-7575 (in California).

Ten

Diabetes
and Diet

Each year over 160,000 people die as a result of diabetes and its complications ranking it fourth among causes of death by disease in the United States. Direct and indirect costs for diabetes are nearly $92 billion annually.[1]

In America alone, more than 14 million people are believed to have diabetes, half of which are undiagnosed. Over 700,000 cases are diagnosed each year. Diabetes is the leading cause of new cases of blindness in ages 20 to 74. Diabetes caused blindness is increasing dramatically up from 5,000 to 12,000 cases each year. Ten percent of all people with diabetes develop some kind of kidney disease. This includes end-stage kidney disease in which a person requires dialysis or a kidney transplant in order to live. Nearly 25% of all dialysis patients are people with diabetes. Diabetes causes approximately 45 percent of all non-traumatic leg and foot amputations in the United States. People with diabetes are 2 to 4 times more likely to have heart disease.

Ischemia of the heart is a factor in 50 to 60 percent of the recorded deaths of adults with diabetes. Hypertension rates are also twice as high among people with diabetes, and the risk of stroke increases sixfold.[2]

Diabetes is an ever-increasing epidemic among affluent, animal-eating peoples of the world and it affects about one out of twenty people in America.

Is diabetes unavoidable, or can we help to prevent it?

Adult-onset diabetes makes up nearly 90 percent of all diabetes in America, and a high percentage of cases can be prevented or cured by following *"The Miracle Diet"* program.[3] Adult onset diabetes (also called Type II) is a result of the amount of animal food and fat in our diet. Lack of proper exercise also contributes to the problem, but the *wrong food* is the *primary problem*.

Childhood diabetes (Type I) may be greatly improved by following *"The Miracle Diet."* The risk of early onset life threatening complications and death can be decreased by basically eating plant foods. For some unknown reason the pancreas does not produce enough insulin in childhood (Type I) diabetes.

Late Research Implicates Milk Protein in cause of Type I Diabetes

It has long been suspected that cows milk proteins are a principal cause of diabetes in children, and a 1992 report in the New England Journal of Medicine adds more support for this explanation. When comparing different countries, the prevalence of insulin-dependent diabetes parallels the consumption of cow's milk. Children who are not exposed to cow's milk products early in life have a dramatically lower risk of diabetes.

In the July 1992 report, researchers from Canada and Finland found evidence that implicated cow's milk in every one of the 142 diabetic children they studied. The culprit appears to be a cow's milk protein, called bovine serum albumin, which differs just enough from human proteins to cause the human body to react by producing antibodies. The antibodies gradually attack and destroy the insulin-producing beta cells of the pancreas.

Everyone of the 142 diabetic children had high levels of antibodies to the cow protein at the time the diabetes was diagnosed. The researchers found that non-diabetic children may have such antibodies but only at low levels.

The form of diabetes which begins in childhood is a leading cause of blindness, and contributes to medical problems including heart disease, kidney problems, and amputations due to poor circulation. The report indicates that the combination of genetic predisposition and cow's milk exposure is the cause of the childhood form of diabetes.

Some diabetes researchers have long suspected milk protein because a segment of it is chemically identical to a protein on the surface of pancreas cells that produce insulin, which regulates blood-sugar levels.

Antibodies produced against the milk protein during the first year of life, the researchers speculate, also attack and destroy the pancreas in a so-called auto-immune reaction, producing diabetes in people whose genetic makeup leaves them vulnerable.

This is good reason for mothers to feed their babies with mother's milk and never use cow's milk or commercial formulas derived from it.[4]

Heredity Not the Primary Factor

Even though in some families the tendency toward diabetes is passed on genetically, making some people more susceptible than others to adult-onset diabetes, heredity is not the primary factor involved. Adult onset diabetes is a different disease than childhood variety. People with adult diabetes usually produce plenty of insulin, and the pancreas sometimes produces twice as much insulin as is produced by normal individuals. The insulin just doesn't work, because it is immobilized by the high fat content in the diet.

Southwest Indians: Their Problem

Before the Southwest Indians began eating white man's food, their diet consisted of beans, squash, corn, prickly pear (a cactus fruit) pods, mesquite bean flour, cholla cactus buds, seeds, oak acorn, and a little meat obtained by hunting.

After World War II, the U.S. government began giving the Indians U.S. surplus commodities, consisting of cheese, lard, butter, peanut butter, and meat. This tax-supported generosity has created a nation of Indian diabetics.

The Indians began to eat a consistently high-fat diet with little complex carbohydrate or fiber. They also abandoned physically demanding activities. When these lifestyle changes were superimposed on a susceptible genetic makeup, the Indians developed a high incidence of obesity and an epidemic of Type II diabetes.

There are now over 250,000 Indian diabetics in Arizona and it is estimated that the annual cost of treating them will rise to two billion dollars by the year 2000. The Pima tribe residing in south central

Arizona has the highest incidence of diabetes in the world. More than 50 percent of all adults over 35 years of age are diabetics. Diabetes in this population has increased over 40 percent in the last 20 years. One half of the Papago Indians who have had diabetes for more than 10 years complain of **impotence.** Tribal chairman Josiah Moore said, "If we don't turn this around, as a nation, in 35-50 years, we're down the tubes."[5]

The Micronesians In Nauru: Their Problem

Diabetes is rare among Asians and Africans, who eat basically plant food. Before World War II Micronesians enjoyed excellent health and a very low incidence of diabetes. The Nauru in Micronesia, once a poor people who are now wealthy, provide a good example of an isolated island society that changed from their native plant diet to an affluent high-fat animal diet after the war. As a result, they developed diabetes and other degenerative diseases.

As they began to eat rich and expensive animal food imported from New Zealand and Australia health deteriorated to the point where one-third of the population over fifteen years of age now suffers from diabetes and the terrible degenerative circulatory diseases that are a result of diabetes. People of Nauru have the second highest rate of diabetes in the world.[6]

THREE CAUSES OF ADULT TYPE II DIABETES
(1) Fats and Oils can Paralyze Insulin

Three components in the affluent animal-eating diet of most Americans and other affluent animal-eating nations cause most adult-onset diabetes. Fats and the oils, which account for 40 to 50 percent of the calorie content of Western diets, act by interfering with insulin activity. The cells of the body become unable to respond to insulin. Amazingly the effect of fats and oils as a major cause of diabetes has been known for more than sixty years.

In 1927, Dr. S. Sweeny fed healthy, young medical students for two days on a diet very high in both animal and vegetable fats then gave them a glucose tolerance test. All of his students showed blood sugar levels high enough to classify them as diabetic.

In another experiment using the same students, before running glucose tolerance tests, Dr. Sweeny fed them simple and complex carbohydrates consisting of sugar, candy, pastry, white bread, baked potatoes, syrup, bananas, rice, and oatmeal. After this high-starch and high-sugar diet was maintained for two days, glucose tolerance tests showed that all of the students were normal, without evidence of diabetes.[7]

(2) Complex Carbohydrates Increase the Power of Insulin
On the other hand, both complex and simple carbohydrates have the opposite effect of fat and oils. Carbohydrates can increase the power of insulin. Anything other than small amounts of sugars should be avoided, because they provide only empty calories. Studies during the past sixty years show that the *lack* of complex carbohydrates contributes to diabetes.[8]

(3) Sixty Grams of Fiber Each Day is Essential
Another problem is the lack of fiber in the average diet. As stated before, there is absolutely NO FIBER in animal flesh, eggs, milk, cheese, or any other animal by-products. White bread, white rice, and other highly refined cereals have had much of the fiber removed. All foods made with white flour and simple sugars—such as cakes, cookies, and pies—are practically devoid of fiber, and sometimes contain more than 50 percent fat.

Fiber, by several mechanisms, slows the absorption into the bloodstream of the products of digestion of simple and complex carbohydrates found in foods. This gradual release of sugars into the bloodstream is believed to be better synchronized with the action of the body's insulin-secreting cells. Just adding more fiber to the diet of a diabetic without changing the fat or carbohydrate content improves the blood sugar levels.[9]

Obesity Contributes to Diabetes
Obesity also contributes to the development of diabetes. Obesity is caused by eating high-fat, low-carbohydrate, low-fiber foods. It appears that in an obese person the tissue cells are less sensitive to the varied actions of insulin, and blood sugar can rise to abnormally high levels.[10]

Diabetes Is Accelerating among Americans

If we are to judge from case studies as well as from the populations we have been able to observe, it appears that the diet described in *"The Miracle Diet"* helps prevent diabetes. Just the opposite is true of the Standard American diet. This disease-promoting lifestyle keeps the diabetic from getting better and helps promote diabetes. This trend has increased to epidemic proportions over the past ninety years among affluent, animal-eating people around the world.

The University of Kentucky is pioneering a program to help people who have been diabetic for as long as thirty years. Researchers start patients out on the Diabetic Association's old diabetic eating program, which includes animal foods high in fats and low in complex carbohydrates. They stabilize them on this diet to find out how much insulin they need. Then they switch them to a plant diet, high in complex carbohydrate, low in fat, and high in fiber. Within three weeks they can, in most cases, take the patients completely off insulin. Blood sugar drops dramatically, even without weight loss.

Researchers report they can get from two-thirds to three-fourths of adult-type diabetics off all insulin or medication; they can get 90 percent off diabetic pills. All of these changes take place by just changing the type of *fuel* that is eaten. Other universities with similar programs report the same results. (This applies only to adult-onset diabetes, not to juvenile-onset diabetes, although experiments show that children with diabetes can benefit in many ways from a diet consisting mainly of plant foods.)[11]

It Has Taken Sixty Years

Just recently the Diabetic Association finally changed its recommended diet from 45 percent carbohydrate to 65 percent carbohydrate. It is now recommending less than 30 percent fat and less than three-hundred milligrams of cholesterol. The Association also now recommends a low-protein diet to preserve kidney function. These guidelines are a step in the right direction, but for the *"Best Possible Health,"* become a plantarian![12]

Eleven

High Blood Pressure: An Epidemic in America

By some estimates, blood pressure problems affect almost half of all Americans. Nearly sixty million people in America suffer from high blood pressure; two-thirds of them are under the age of sixty-five.[1] But according to an increasing number of researchers, most cases of high blood pressure can be prevented.

Epidemiological studies from around the world show that billions of people in Asian and African countries who eat plant foods as their major source of calories hardly ever develop high blood pressure (hypertension). Only in countries where people eat animals and animal-by-products and high amounts of man-made vegetable fats do they seem to suffer from hypertension.

High blood pressure is not a disease in itself. Basically, it is only a *sign* of disease. World-renowned researchers say that a reading of 110/70 or less is ideal, and nearly all people who eat mostly plant food seldom exceed that ideal blood pressure, even into advanced age. In the Western world we have been told to expect our blood pressure to rise as we grow older. However this only happens when people eat rich animal food throughout their lifetime as the main source of calories.[2]

What Causes High Pressure?

Dr. John A. McDougall, well-known author and world-wide researcher on diet and health, put it this way. . . .

"If you get excited, your heart, the pump, pumps harder and the pressure in the system goes up," he explains. "If you eat added salt, the salt will cause water to accumulate in the body, especially in about twenty percent of the people, and this added water in the blood pumping system causes the pressure to go up.

"If you eat high amounts of fat as we do in America, both animal and added vegetable fat, the fat causes the blood to sludge, raising the pressure in the pumping system.

"Animal food also causes spasms to occur in the tiny blood vessels in the body, causing the pumping pressure to go up because of the contractions in the blood vessels.

"Eating animal food causes cholesterol to accumulate in our blood vessels, which in turn causes plaquing and hardening of the arteries. The arteries become inflexible from artery disease, which turns up the pressure in the pumping system."

Dr. McDougall points out that the process is like "placing your finger over the end of your garden hose so that you would make more pressure in the water pumping system when you want to squirt a flower twenty feet from you. This is what high blood pressure is; all your little hoses are squeezed. There is no place for the blood to go, and the blood pressure in your pumping system goes up."

McDougall explains that the body's "hoses," or blood vessels are squeezed by "(1) atherosclerosis; (2) blood sludging that occurs after a fatty meal; and, (3) the spasms that occur as a result of fat and animal food. There just isn't any place for the blood to go. *The pressure goes up.* This gives us a *sign* that there is trouble in the pumping system. The blood vessels are sick and the circulation is in trouble. The way that most medical people deal with this is they make the sign go away. Nothing is done to improve the health of the arteries, and in many cases medicine makes the arteries worse.

"When you take someone and lower his or her blood pressure, as a treatment of high blood pressure, instead of dealing with the sludged, plugged, rotten arteries it results in failure, and that's what the treatment of high blood pressure with drugs is doing.

"Beta Blockers stop the activity of adrenalin on the heart and in effect they weaken the pump. They raise triglycerides and they lower the good kind of cholesterol. It is believed they raise the chances of dying of heart disease because of these factors.

"Diuretic drugs increase your cholesterol and triglycerides, make you more diabetic, and raise your uric acid. When you take two groups of people, one treated with diuretics and the other not, those treated with diuretics have an increased risk of dying of heart disease. In fact those on diuretics have twice the risk of dying a *sudden death*.

"Another way to lower blood pressure is to dilate the blood vessels. Drugs that dilate blood vessels only seem to dilate healthy blood vessels and do nothing to improve the health of the arteries.

"This may shock you, but it is the truth, verified by a great deal of scientific data. Patients with diastolic blood pressures of 104 will not receive appreciable benefit from lowering their blood pressure with medication. That's what the studies consistently show. We have people in our society who have diastolic blood pressure of 85, 90, 95, and 100 and they are the ones who are being treated with blood pressure pills.

"People do not die of high blood pressure. They die of rotten arteries. We need to make the arteries stronger and healthier by treating the cause. Diseased arteries are fragile and will break under any level of pressure. When you look at healthy arteries they are very strong. Weight lifters' blood pressure goes up to 450/350 and does not hurt even one blood vessel.

"In animal experiments where they attached them to machines and raised their blood pressure into the thousands of millimeters of pressure, not a single healthy blood vessel breaks. Strong blood vessels do not break under any pressure we might cause in our body, but rotten blood vessels break under any pressure.

"High blood pressure is not the disease, it is only a *sign* of disease. When we deal with the cause, the sign gets better and the pressure comes down.

"Almost anybody can lower his or her blood pressure to normal who changes to a starch-based diet with vegetables and fruits. Some have to lower their salt intake, and getting some exercise helps too. Most people on medication can get off medication and have a normal pressure. Now the shocking part of it is that it happens in only about two days. It's amazing how quickly the body corrects itself after you stop sludging your blood with fatty meals."[3]

A plant-based diet seems to be the best solution to correct most cases of elevated blood pressure.

Watch the Salt!

For years doctors believed that salt was a major factor in high blood pressure, but researchers now say that only about 20 percent of all people are sensitive to salt.

Salt does contribute to hypertension, but it is only one of the causes. Lowering fat intake to 10 percent or less, severely restricting animal food, eating mostly complex carbohydrates, and restricting salt intake to what is in plant foods will bring most people with hypertension into a normal blood pressure range within a few days or weeks.[4]

Your body needs some salt, but the natural salt present in a variety of plant foods more than suffices for most people. The National Research Council reports that 500 milligrams (1/4 teaspoon) of sodium a day is adequate for practically all adults. The National Academy of Sciences limits maximum salt intake to no more than 2400 milligrams of sodium per day. The average American eats from five to fifteen thousand milligrams of sodium per day which is ten to thirty times the body's needs.[5]

Higher blood pressure isn't the only result of too much salt. Salt can upset your natural water/salt balance, forcing the body to hold onto extra water. Just a little salt can add extra pounds of retained water in your body. Your heart has to work harder because your tissues are flooded in the spaces between the blood capillaries. Salt-caused edema (swelling) can cut down your capillary blood oxygen transfer to the cells between the capillaries. Some researchers believe that edema creates a host of circulatory problems, including arthritis, reduced visual, auditory, and tactile sensations and joint stiffness. Salt can also create extra pressure against the vessel walls.[6]

High Blood Pressure Is Curable with a Plant Diet

World-renowned Dr. Walter Kempner of Duke University has shown in his on-going studies for more than forty years that high blood pressure can be lowered dramatically by diet alone. Interestingly enough, the diet he uses is strictly plant food. It is basically The Miracle Diet program. Kempner's studies proved that a diet of rice, fruit, and fruit juices cures high blood pressure and many other health problems in most cases. These studies have been well documented in the scientific medical literature for more than four decades. Even extreme cases of high blood pressure have been cured in 60 percent of the cases.[7]

Medication Is Not the Answer

Medications are not the answer. There are just too many side effects from high blood pressure drugs. Scientists tell us that many of the drugs, especially the thiazide diuretics, have been shown to cause irregular heart rhythm. These drugs have also been shown to reduce blood potassium.

In addition to irregular heartbeats, thiazide diuretics can have adverse effects on metabolism. Thiazides can also contribute to elevated levels of both blood sugar and uric acid, leading to diabetes and gout. Thiazides also seem to raise the blood cholesterol and triglyceride levels in the blood.

It is well documented in many studies that cholesterol causes heart disease. Other studies show that the death rate is higher among people with mild high blood pressure who are on blood pressure pills as compared to people with mild high blood pressure using no medication at all.[8]

What Can You Do?

If you are on medication for high blood pressure, you will need to monitor your blood pressure carefully when you change to *"The Miracle Diet."* Consult with your medical practitioner about cutting down on your medication as your pressure comes down.

Twelve

Antioxidants:
Nature's Cancer Killers
Fight Free Radicals

Dr. Julian Whitaker, M.D., noted author and nutritionist says, "Don't look now, but your house is burning down. Not that multi-room structure you live in, but your body—it is burning down. Your body has been on a slow burn since your birth, and now you can either accelerate its destruction or slow it down. Frankly, the latter option seems preferable.

"Your body is constantly being damaged by free radicals, ions which are naturally produced by the oxidation of food. It is as if the fire in your home fireplace kept spurting out embers that burn holes in the rugs and furniture and could set the whole place ablaze.

"Free radicals, the embers of food combustion, are extremely toxic to cell membranes, proteins, and even the DNA of your chromosomes. They are now considered to be a major cause of aging and of most of our degenerative diseases, including heart disease, cancer, multiple sclerosis, and arthritis, to mention a few.

"Dr. Denhan Harman first articulated the free radical theory of aging and disease in 1959. Like any new theory, it has taken a while to catch on, but has been validated and significantly expanded, particularly over the last five years. Some of the most exciting research of this century concerns how free radicals are produced, how they damage the body, and what the body does to protect itself from this damage."[1]

Try this Test

Hold one of your hands out in front of you palm down. Next, using your other hand, pinch and lift the skin on the back of your outstretched hand. When you let go, does your skin quickly snap back into place? Is it flat or smooth? Or does it just sort of slump back into place?

When we are young, our skin snaps briskly back, but as we age, our skin loses its elasticity. It begins to wrinkle. Age spots appear. Why? Because the oxygen in the air around us damages our skin. You can see evidence of similar damage everywhere—from the rust that forms on an old car to the windshield wiper blades that you need to replace because they have become dry, brittle, and hard.

We call this process oxidation. Oxygen reacts with the molecules in these materials—the iron in the car, the rubber in the wiper, the skin on your hand. The oxygen molecule loses an electron to become a free radical that produces the damaging effects of rust or aging skin. So powerful is this process that, over time, free radicals even will break down concrete.

Because they are so reactive, free radicals will attack almost any material including the more than 75 trillion cells in the human body. In the process, they will damage the outer cell membrane, opening the door for a variety of ailments.

Free radicals are suspects in more than 60 human diseases, ranging from cancer of the lungs, mouth, throat, stomach, bladder, and rectum, to heart disease. Free radicals cause veins and capillaries to become brittle with age. A decade-long study found that they are what makes cholesterol cling to the sides of arteries.

Try this Experiment

Cut an apple in half. Dip half the apple in orange juice. Leave the other half the way it is. Wait for a half hour. You'll notice that half of the apple has turned brown as a result of free radical damage caused by contact with oxygen in the air. The other half of the apple-the part dipped in orange juice will still be crisp and white.

Why the difference? An antioxidant has saved the half of the apple dipped in orange juice. Antioxidants are unique substances that counteract the damaging effects of free radical oxygen molecules. They do this by giving up an electron so that the oxygen returns to its less reactive and more stable formation. One such antioxidant is vitamin C, found in orange juice. By coating the apple with vitamin C, you created a shield against free radical damage.

This process has important consequences for human health. It is the reason the main antioxidants in the human diet (vitamins C and E, beta carotene, and selenium) are some of the brightest stars in today's nutritional scientific research.

Health Professionals Jumping on
Antioxidant Bandwagon

Now, health professionals, who denied the value of such food components a few years ago, have jumped on the antioxidant bandwagon. Newsweek quoted a Harvard physician as saying, "until very recently, it was taught that everyone in this country gets enough vitamins . . . I think we have proof that this isn't true. I think the scientific community has realized this is a very important area of research."

The research, in turn, is bearing out what many biochemists have suspected for some time—there are many benefits from a diet high in plant-food nutrients. Harvard University, the University of California-San Diego, the University of California-Berkeley, the University of Alabama, and the National Cancer Institute, among others, have conducted studies confirming that antioxidants found in plant foods play a powerful role in human health.

One study involving 120,000 men and women during an eight year period showed that an increased intake of vitamin E reduced the risk of heart disease by about 40%. A Harvard University study found beta carotene reduced the risk of heart attack among men with a history of heart disease.[2]

To reap these benefits, many people are turning to a plant-centered diet, changing their lifestyles and eating patterns to benefit from an antioxidant-rich diet of plants.

Avoid the Ravages of Free Radicals

The best way to improve your chances of avoiding the ravages of free radicals and remaining healthy is through a change in fuel, a plant-centered diet in place of your present animal-centered diet. Center your food on the *five basic starches* supplemented with a wide variety of green and yellow vegetables as well as fruit.

"The US Department of Agriculture's Food Guide Pyramid of 1992 tells us to get up to 85% of our calories from plant sources." Animal Food and added Fats are limited to little or none if you want to be attractive, lean and healthy.

The National Cancer Institute is now recommending that we eat five servings of green and yellow vegetables each day along with three servings of fruit. These foods are naturally high in antioxidant nutrients. Spinach, cabbage, broccoli, brussell sprouts, collard greens, kale, turnip greens, and many other green leafy vegetables also have significant amounts of the antioxidant nutrients on which researchers are focusing.

Many People are Changing

Many people are listening to this advice and changing their diets and the quality of their lives is improving. Finally, the modern American diet, forced by rising rates of cancer, diabetes, osteoporosis, heart disease and pushed by spiraling health care costs, is taking a turn for the better. If you're wondering if the benefits of making the change are worth it, try this: Hold one of your hands in front of you, palm down. . . .

Thirteen

Millions Starve
So We Can Eat Meat

Let's consider what we can do for humanity if we adopt *"The Miracle Diet"* lifestyle. Can we feel comfortable when tens of thousands of children starve to death on this earth everyday? Literally tens of millions of our fellow human beings starve to death each year.

John Robbins' classic book, *Diet For a New America,* helps us understand the consequences of our overwhelming desire to consume animals in our affluent society. "The livestock population of the United States today consumes enough grain and soybeans to feed over five times the entire human population of the country. We feed these animals over 80% of the corn we grow and over 95% of the oats." [1]

He says: "It is hard to grasp how immensely wasteful is a meat-oriented diet-style. By cycling our grain through livestock, we end up with only 10% as many calories available to feed human mouths as would be available if we ate the grain directly."

"Less than half of the harvested agricultural acreage in the United States is used to grow food for people. Most of it is used to grow livestock feed. For every sixteen pounds of grain and soybeans fed to beef cattle we get back only one pound as meat on our plates."[2]

In Robbins' well-documented book, he reveals more startling and heart-rending conditions. "Forty thousand children starve to death on this planet every day. To supply food for a year for one person with a meat habit requires three-and-a-quarter acres. To supply food for a year for one pure vegetarian requires only one-sixth of an acre. In other words, a given acreage can feed twenty times as many people eating a pure vegetarian diet-style as it could people eating the standard American diet-style."[3]

Can we ignore the needs of humanity? Think of the good we could accomplish by being examples to the rest of the world as we lead out in changing our eating habits and thus provide more food to the starving millions.

Shocking Statistics!

John Robbins continues to provide us with mind-boggling information: "By cycling our grain through livestock, we not only waste 90 percent of its protein; in addition we sadly waste 96 percent of its calories, 100 percent of its fiber, and 100 percent of its carbohydrates. [4] The world's cattle alone, not to mention pigs and chickens, consume a quantity of food equal to the caloric needs of 8.7 billion people-nearly double the entire population of the planet. According to Department of Agriculture statistics, one acre of land can grow 20,000 pounds of potatoes. That same acre of land, if used to grow cattle-feed, can produce less than 165 pounds of beef."[5]

A Child Starves Every Two Seconds

Robbins then makes this comment: "In a world in which a child dies of starvation every two seconds, an agricultural system designed to feed our meat habit is a blasphemy. Yet it continues, because we continue to support it. As long as enough people continue to purchase their products they will have the resources to fight reforms, pump millions of dollars of educational propaganda into our schools, and defend themselves against medical and ethical truths."[6]

We Are Losing Our Topsoil

There are many more aspects to be considered such as losing our topsoil to erosion. John Robbins attributes much of the loss of our topsoil to the "hyped-up demands we require to feed huge numbers of livestock." Robbins says that "two hundred years ago, most of America's croplands had at least 21 inches of topsoil. Today, most of it is down to around six inches of topsoil, and the rate of topsoil loss is accelerating." He adds: "Pure vegetarian food choices make less than 5% of the demand on the soil as meat-oriented choices."[7]

Much of the deforestation in the United States appears to be the result of feeding livestock. More and more, beef used in North

America comes from Central and South America, and these countries are clearing tropical rain forests to make pasture land for these cattle. Robbins says, "These tropical rain forests are among the world's most precious natural resources. Amounting to only 30 percent of the earth's forests, containing 80 percent of all land vegetation, and accounting for a substantial percentage of the earth's oxygen supplies."[8]

Water Shortages

Water shortages in the United States are creating greater concerns each year. Consider a few statements by John Robbins:

(1) "Over half the total amount of water consumed in the U.S. goes to irrigate land growing feed and fodder for livestock. Enormous additional quantities of water must also be used to wash away the animals excrement. It would be hard to design a less water efficient diet-style than the one we come to think of as normal."

(2) "To produce a single pound of meat takes an average of 2,500 gallons of water—as much as a typical family uses for all its combined household purposes in a month."

(3) "To produce a day's food for one meat-eater takes 4,000 gallons; for a pure vegetarian, only 300 gallons."

(4) "It takes up to a hundred times more water to produce a pound of meat as it does to produce a pound of wheat."

(5) "If the cost of water needed to produce a pound of meat were not subsidized by government taxes, the cheapest hamburger meat would cost more than $35 a pound."[9]

Livestock Manure Polluting Our Water

These are only a few statements showing the connection between water waste and our animal appetites in America. Let's consider the pollution to our water supplies. John Robbins continues,

(1) "Fifty years ago, most of the manure from livestock returned to enrich the soil. But today, with huge numbers of animals concentrated in feedlots, confinement buildings, and other factory farm locations, there is no economically feasible way to return their wastes to the soil. As a result there is a continuing decline in soil humus and soil fertility, an ever increasing dependence on chemical fertilizers and pesticides, and an accelerating loss of topsoil."

(2) "Sadly, instead of being returned to the soil, the wastes from today's animals often end up in our water."

(3) "Every 24 hours, the animals destined for America's dinner table produce 20 billion pounds of waste."

(4) "The livestock of the United States produce twenty times as much excrements as the entire human population of the country! Over a billion tons a year comes from confinement operations from which it cannot be recycled."

(5) "Animal wastes account for more than ten times as much water pollution as the total amount attributable to the entire human population."

(6) "One cow produces as much waste as 16 humans. With 20,000 animals in our pens, we have a problem equal to a city of 320,000 people."[10]

John Robbins details many more reasons why a plantarian lifestyle is of great value aside from personal and public health reasons. He discusses the conditions of animals on modern factory farms and the subject of compassion as it affects our total outlook on life here on earth. I recommend that you read *Diet For a New America* to help you become aware of all the consequences of eating animals as your major intake of calories.

"Teaching" The "New Four Food Groups"

The Physicians Committee for Responsible Medicine said the methods of teaching Americans good nutrition should be changed to reflect the mounting evidence that diets high in fat and low in fiber increase the risk of degenerative disease.

A 1988 study by the surgeon general said diet-related diseases account for at least 68% of all deaths in the United States.

The Physicians Committee for Responsible Medicine report said nutritional requirements, including protein, zinc, calcium and iron, can be met on a plant-based diet, pointing out that the average American eats two to five times as much protein as needed. They said the **"New Four Food Groups"** does not rely on any admonition to use particular foods in moderation, since all of the foods in this guideline can be consumed without restrictions.[11]

Their report was critical of the government's call on Americans to cut back—but not omit foods high in cholesterol and fat. It went on to say that previous recommendations have protected the image of certain foods and "promoted the health of food industries."

They said the **"New Four Food Groups"** would encourage Americans to perceive cereals (whole grains), legumes, vegetables and fruit as essential, and milk or a piece of meat as a non-essential extra.[12]

Dr. Neal D. Barnard, M.D. is Associate Director for Behavioral Studies at the Institute for Disease Prevention of George Washington University School of Medicine, where he has conducted research into programs that help change eating habits.

The *Power of Your Plate* and his latest book *Food for Life* are available in most bookstores or from the Physicians Committee for Responsible Medicine, P.O. Box 6322, Washington, D.C. 20016.

Athletic Competition and Carbo-loading

Marathon runners, distance cyclists, swimmers, and other athletes use the term, "carbo-loading" which means storing carbohydrate for energy in the liver before competition. Many world records have been broken on the athletic field by plantarians during the last few years. David Scott, the world's triathlete during the 80's eats a plant-based diet. Other athletes, whose names you may recognize are eating a plantarian diet—Edwin Moses, the great 1976 and 1984 Olympic Gold Medal hurdler, Murray Rose, the Olympic Gold Medal swimmer considered by many to be the greatest swimmer of all time, Paavo Nurmi, the distance runner who won nine Olympic Gold and Silver medals and set 20 world records, James and Jonathan de Donato, who jointly hold the world's record for distance butterfly stroke swimming, and numerous others could be mentioned. It's no surprise that endurance tests with a variety of diets show the superiority of a plant-centered diet.[13-15]

Superior Health of Seventh-Day Adventists

Seventh-Day Adventists are the best example of any major religious group in America as far as nutrition and health is concerned. JAMA, the Journal of the American Medical Association, published two studies in the first six months of 1992, that statistically prove that Seventh-Day Adventists live longer than the general population of Americans.

About half of the Seventh-Day Adventists in California follow a lacto-ovo vegetarian diet (plant food plus milk and eggs). and have an age-adjusted prostate cancer mortality rate that is only 30 percent that of the general population.[16] There is a statistically significant decreased risk of cancer for men with relatively higher consumption of legumes and citrus fruit, and an increased risk seen for those with a higher total consumption of meat products, particularly fish. Seventh-Day Adventists have significantly lower overall rates of mortality from most major chronic diseases, including coronary artery disease and cancers, compared to the general American population.[17]

In a 1985 medical study on diabetes, Dr. David Snowden of the University of Minnesota and Dr. Roland Phillips of Loma Linda University collected data on 25,698 Seventh-Day Adventists over a 21 year period. They found that plant eaters were significantly less likely to die from diabetes-related causes than meat eaters.[18]

William P. Castelli, M.D., Director of the Framingham Heart Study, the longest running heart study in the world, offers the Seventh-Day Adventists as an example of quality of life as well as longevity. He says, "Their philosophy calls for a vegetarian (and therefore low cholesterol) diet, regular exercise and abstention from alcohol, caffeine and tobacco products." Dr. Castelli points out that Seventh-Day Adventist men outlive other Americans by seven years, and women by five years. He goes on to state that "they have only 15 percent of our heart-attack rate and 40 percent of our cancer rate.[19]

Most Seventh-Day Adventists are not total plantarians. Many Adventists admit they could and should follow an even better diet with much less fat and fewer eggs and dairy products. This would most likely give them an even more impressive record of health and longevity. However, Seventh-Day Adventists probably put more emphasis on nutrition than any other religious group in America. They are a good example of a people who teach the value of nutrition in obtaining better health, quality of life and longevity.

Mormons and Health

The Mormon Religion has a code of health called the Word of Wisdom. Their philosophy calls for abstention from tobacco, alcohol, tea and coffee as well as the following food health code:

">. . . all wholesome herbs [**plants**] God hath ordained for the constitution, nature, and use of man—every herb [**plant**] in the season thereof, and every fruit in the season thereof; all these to be used with prudence and thanksgiving.

"Yea, *flesh* also of *beasts [animals]* and of the *fowls* of the air, . . . are to be used *sparingly*; . . . *they* should *not* be used, *only* in times of *winter*, or of *cold*, or *famine*.

"All *grain* is ordained for the use of *man* and of beasts, to be the *staff of life*, not only for man but for the *beasts* of the field, and the *fowls* of heaven, and all *wild animals* that run or creep on earth; and *these [beasts, fowls, and wild animals]* hath God made for the use of man *only* in times of *famine* and excess of *hunger*.

"*All grain* is good for the *food* of *man*; as also the *fruit* of the vine; that which yieldeth fruit, whether *in* the ground or *above* the ground—." [20] (emphasis added)

Dictionary Defines:
"*Staff of life*" as a "**staple of diet.**"
"*Staple*" is defined as "the sustaining or **principal element; something used, needed, or enjoyed constantly.**"
and "*Sparingly*" means "barely, slightly, meagerly or sparsely."

In interviews most Mormons admit they eat meat, chicken and fish on a regular basis, but many say they need to change. Former Mormon Church President Ezra Taft Benson, (who also served as The United States Secretary of Agriculture from 1953 to 1961), perhaps said it best, "We are an overfed and undernourished nation, digging an early grave with our teeth, and lacking the energy that could be ours. . . . We need a generation of people who eat in a healthier manner." [21]

Some Tough Questions

We ask ourselves, "Are we our brothers keeper?" Are we responsible for the earth? Are we willing to change so that our posterity has better health and a better place to live? It is exciting to see the change taking place in America as more and more people are becoming aware of the importance of the *"Best Possible Health"* by eating a plant-centered diet.

Fourteen

Change: Making It All Work With Diet and Exercise

All plant food can be eaten singly or in any combination. Starches are the core of The Miracle Diet program. Starches (grains, rice, corn, legumes) also potatoes and other vegetables take the place of animal flesh and animal-foods, including animal by-products such as milk, cheese, sour cream, cottage cheese, ice cream and eggs.

Complex Carbohydrates

Since starches are made up mostly of complex carbohydrates, they take longer to metabolize. In general, the more unrefined the carbohydrate, the longer it takes for the body to break it down for use as a fuel for energy. Complex carbohydrates release a slow, constant stream of glucose into the bloodstream, approximately two calories per minute. This seems to be the optimal rate for the body's energy demands. Only carbohydrates burn 100 percent clean in the process of converting into energy.[1]

The Five Basic Starches

There are five common starch foods:

(1) **GRAINS**, such as WHEAT, OATS, BARLEY, and RYE. At least two of these grains should be used daily.

(2) **BROWN RICE** (another basic grain.)

(3) **CORN**, a starch, is really another grain. It is a great food, and for millennia whole cultures have used it as their basic source of calories.

(4) **BEANS**, another starch, provide more and better protein than meat.

(5) **POTATOES,** including sweet potatoes, can be eaten three times a day if desired. They'll keep you healthy.

These starch foods have just the right amount of protein, carbohydrate, fat, and fiber for the optimum needs of the body. Beans, peas, and lentils are high in protein and therefore should be limited to three or four times a week, if you eat more than one cup a day.

With starch as your foundation, add various vegetables of your choice. Every day eat a raw vegetable salad filled with lots of different vegetables, not just lettuce. Always keep a variety of cut-up vegetables in the refrigerator, and use them at meals or snacks instead of salads. Each day you can also eat some cooked green or yellow vegetables. Potatoes, white or sweet, can be eaten every day if you like them. White potatoes are very low in fat (1 percent), the lowest of any commonly used vegetable. I am convinced that potatoes are probably the finest all-around basic food for the *"Best Possible Health,"* and most children like potatoes, too. Rice runs a close second as an outstanding basic food for man.

Fruit is a Great Dessert

Three fruits a day add to the enjoyment of *"The Miracle Diet."* Any type of fruit may be eaten. If your triglyceride level is over 200, you might be better off limiting your fruits to three or fewer per day. If your triglycerides are 100 or less, you could eat more, but not in place of your starches. If you desire maximum weight loss eat only 2 fruits per day. Simple carbohydrates (sugars) have a tendency to increase blood triglycerides—which means more free fat is flowing in your bloodstream. Because fruits are high in sugar, they can cause excess blood fats in some people.

All "Essential Amino Acids" and "Essential Fats" Are in *"The Miracle Diet"*

An all plant diet gives you all the essential vitamins, minerals, and fiber you require. You will also get all the essential amino acids as well as linoleic acid, a very important essential fat—one the body doesn't manufacture. Just three and one-half ounces of oatmeal every day supplies you with all the linoleic acid you need. Your need for essential fat is less than 2% of calories in your diet. It is nearly impossible to have a deficiency in essential fat in adults.

Amazingly, essential fats are synthesized only by plants, not by animals. Plant foods, even those low in fat, provide plenty of essential fat for humans.[2-3]

What About Vitamin B 12?

If you are pregnant or nursing, or if you follow this program strictly for more than three years, then take at least 5 micrograms supplemental vitamin B12 each day.

Eat Three Full Meals Each Day—and Snacks

Be sure to eat at least three full meals every day. Don't stay hungry between meals. Eat snacks as long as they are made of plant food without any added fats or oils. Try whole wheat bread, plain or toasted, air-popped popcorn, or plain corn tortillas baked in a pre-heated oven for thirty minutes at 350°. You can now buy baked no-added-fat corn chips like Tostitos, by Frito-Lay, Inc. and other brands found in health food and grocery stores. There are a number of no-fat-added pretzels and fat-free potato chips like Louise's and other brands.

Pita or pocket bread usually has no added fat. It's a good snack that can be filled with vegetables or toasted and eaten with a little jam. Some store-purchased whole wheat bread has a minimal amount of oil, sweetening, and salt; eat only the best 100 percent whole wheat bread you can find, or better still, make your own. Read labels carefully. Avoid a diet of white bread, white rice, refined cereals, and any other fiber-deficient foods.

For maximum weight loss hold back on all flour products such as bread, pretzels, and bagels. Flour products are ground fine and will increase the absorption of calories, slowing down weight loss.

Secret of Staying On and Enjoying the Diet

The secret to staying on The Miracle Diet program is to have basic foods cooked and in the refrigerator ready to heat up or eat cold at a moment's notice. You can bake several potatoes in the oven and store them in the refrigerator. Cook one cup of brown rice in two and one-half cups of boiling water and simmer on low for forty-five minutes or until the water is gone, then store in the refrigerator. You can buy an inexpensive automatic rice cooker. Just add water and rice and turn it on. It turns off automatically. You'll love it. Cook four or five cups of dry pinto beans (or whatever kind of beans you prefer) and freeze part of them in small containers for quick snacks or full meals. Cook whole wheat pasta in advance and store it in the refrigerator. Cook plenty of pasta sauce in advance and freeze part of it. It's good on brown rice, too. You can buy fat-free pasta sauce, it's good. Look for it in health food stores or supermarkets.

Potatoes are very Versatile

Potatoes can be fixed in so many different ways: baked in the microwave (six minutes for one, ten minutes for two, fifteen minutes for four), boiled, mashed, or baked in a conventional oven. No-oil frozen hash brown potatoes are great cooked in a non-stick pan. Best of all are oven-baked French fries sprinkled with onion and garlic powder and a little paprika-with no oil or salt. They're ready to eat in half an hour! (Boil the potatoes in their jackets until they are barely tender; cool in the refrigerator. Peel and cut into large French fries, sprinkle with onion and garlic powder and paprika. Put on a non-stick baking sheet and bake in a 400° oven for about 30 minutes.)

Have Vegetable Stew (Soup) on Hand

Vegetable stew (soup) tastes good for any meal or snack and has the perfect ingredients to keep your body healthy. This vegetable stew is wonderful eaten with plenty of whole wheat bread or corn chips.

Use a 6-quart pan; make plenty, because it stores well. Freeze some, and keep some in the refrigerator so that you always have something good to eat when you get hungry. You can reheat it quickly in the microwave or on top of the stove.

4 potatoes, cut in medium-sized chunks
1 48 oz. can tomato juice
4 medium onions, sliced small
1 28 oz. can tomatoes
4 large stalks of celery, sliced

1/2 cup sliced frozen okra, frozen broccoli, or both
4 large carrots, sliced
1/4 teaspoon pepper, dash of red pepper
1/2 cup frozen corn
1/2 teaspoon Mrs. Dash-herbs
1 cup pearled barley
1/2 teaspoon dill weed

In a saucepan add the can of tomato juice to the cut vegetables. Add the can of tomatoes, and cut up the tomatoes. Add 1 cup of water. Bring to a boil. Add seasonings. Simmer over medium-low heat about 30 to 45 minutes. Do not overcook. The carrots should be crunchy. Cook the barley separately and add about 15 minutes before end of cooking time. Add 1/2 cup of corn in the last 3 minutes of cooking time. You may want to use 1 cup of cooked brown rice or broken up whole-wheat spaghetti as options in place of the barley.

Helpful hints: Other vegetables may be used in addition to or in place of the ones listed above. Try 1/2 cup of frozen peas, chopped spinach, sliced mushrooms, or one green pepper added during the last 4 minutes of cooking time.

Bag Lots of Raw Vegetables

Cut up raw celery, carrots, broccoli, cauliflower, purple cabbage, green onions, radishes, and any other raw vegetables you like; refrigerate in individual plastic bags. You'll always have something ready to eat for snacks or use as your raw vegetables at mealtime instead of taking the time to make a salad. When you eat them this way you won't need a salad dressing! Try using Fat-Free salad dressings as a dip for your raw vegetables.

The Simple Way to Eat

If you don't like spending much time cooking and still want to enjoy the ***"Best Possible Health,"*** just learn to enjoy the starches plain. Brown rice is delicious warmed up with only a little pepper as spice; try a little red pepper for variety. Brown rice is wonderful served cold with sliced bananas, applesauce, or other fresh fruits. You can add some cinnamon or nutmeg to make it even better. Brown rice is a perfect food and has a mild nutty flavor all by itself.

Potatoes are quick and easy to fix any time. A bowl of cooked frozen corn takes three minutes and is always delicious. Home-cooked beans can be heated up quickly any time and provide great nutrition (use only every other day, or no more than one cup per day). Read labels on canned beans—many have no added fat and some no salt. There are several good brands of fat-free canned re-fried beans. They are great for sandwiches, tostados, bean nachos, etc. Peas are like beans or lentils; they are high in protein and should be used only every other day, or no more than one cup per day. Potatoes (white or sweet), brown rice, corn, beans, peas, and whole wheat pasta take the place of meat, fish, chicken, or any animal product in your diet.

Less Cleanup Time

It is so much easier to cook plant food in place of animal food, with no fats popping all over your stove and kitchen to clean up. The dishes and pans clean up so easily when no grease coats them. Meals can be served in much less time, and the whole kitchen can be cleaned up much faster and easier. Plus you'll need no Draino because there will be no grease build-up in your drain.

If you enjoy cooking, you can make it just as fancy as you like. Try some of the recipes in this book, make up your own, or convert your favorite recipes to eliminate the fats, sugars, and salt. Egg yolks should not be used, but egg whites can be used in your recipes. If a recipe calls for one egg, use two egg whites as a substitution for the whole egg. A great non-animal substitute is Egg Replacer: ENER-G found in health food stores.

An Easy Day's Menu

BREAKFAST: Make a dry mix of oatmeal and wheat cereal. I use a mixture of Wheatena, oatmeal, and oat bran, equal parts of each mixed dry and stored in a plastic container with a cover. Make up enough to last a week or more.

To prepare, fill a three-quart pan with two quarts of water. Bring to a boil. Add two cups of dry mix to the boiling water. Stir and turn the heat to medium or medium-low. After the cereal cooks a few minutes, add more water to keep it from getting too thick. Cook for thirty minutes or longer, if desired; it becomes smoother as it cooks longer. The cereal provides about two quarts of delicious, fiber-rich food and is the perfect combination of protein, complex carbohydrate, and has little fat.

I recommend as much as one quart every morning. It sounds like a lot of food, but you need lots of natural grains that are high in nutrition and fiber to start the day right. If you are still hungry, eat an orange, banana, or other fruit to top off your perfect breakfast. Breakfast should be your largest meal of the day, because you have gone for hours without eating.

Note: If you like milk on your cereal, you can now find fat-free rice milk or fat-free soy milk in health food stores or in some super markets. Fred Meyer Superstores, a western chain, carries a wonderful line of Health Foods, grains, beans, whole grain cereals, rice, corn, etc.

LUNCH: Vegetable stew or soup, whole wheat bread, raw vegetables or a salad and a fruit of your choice make a great lunch.

The best part of this lunch is that you can heat the stew or soup, put it in a vacuum bottle, and take it with you to work. If you have a microwave oven at your work-place, you can heat it there.

Whole wheat pita bread filled with salad vegetables also makes a great lunch, or try a tomato and lettuce sandwich with raw vegetables and some fruit. There are endless variations: try a couple of cooked cold potatoes with whole wheat bread and an apple—it also makes a good lunch.

DINNER: Try one or more baked potatoes, or brown rice, or both; a large vegetable salad or five or six different raw vegetables and two or more slices of 100 percent whole wheat bread.

You can add a cooked yellow or green vegetable to your dinner if you like. Beans, corn, or whole wheat pasta can be substituted as your main entree starch. Fruit is always good and easy to fix for dessert. There are many variations and combinations of the correct health-supporting foods. Just use a little ingenuity and imagination.

You will enjoy the added energy as your excess weight goes away. You will see a marked improvement in your health and appearance as you become leaner and stronger in only fourteen days after you exchange your animal entrees for starches.

Your body will begin to heal itself within hours after you adopt this diet for the *"Best Possible Health."* You'll enjoy health and strength because you will have changed your eating habits to follow nature's law of health. You will no longer create disease in your arteries by eating killer cholesterol-laden animals and their by-products. At last, you will be free of rich foods that can make you sick.

Commitment and Self-discipline

Yes, it takes commitment and self-discipline to change your lifestyle to a healthier, leaner future. It takes self-discipline to overcome addictions of any kind, whether it is to tobacco, alcohol, drugs or to food. Is it possible animal foods are addicting, too? After fourteen days of eating mostly plant food, you will feel so much better that you'll wonder why you didn't see the wisdom of it all a long time ago.

How Much Exercise?

Once you're eating the best foods, top off your health program with a good exercise program! Start with five to ten minutes of stretching exercises. This increases overall health, vigor, and agility. Muscles have a tendency to tighten up as we grow older, especially after a period of inactivity. Your whole day will be more enjoyable and relaxing if you do stretching exercises each morning just after you wake up. If you have had a tense day, stretching for two minutes before you go to bed at night will help you relax.

One of the healthiest exercises is walking, although any exercise that uses the long leg muscles for a sustained period of time is great. The calves of your legs act as powerful pumps to move the blood back up to your heart.

Walking and other long-leg exercises build additional blood vessels in the legs, bypassing old damaged vessels like varicose veins and stimulating healthy vessels to carry more life-giving blood to the legs and feet.

It might require a period of building up slowly, but walking vigorously for thirty to forty minutes, at least four times each week, will give you the minimum amount of aerobic training. If you want additional exercise, walk briskly six times per week or walk twice a day four days a week.

If you enjoy sports and more vigorous aerobic training, try jogging, running, handball, racketball, squash, basketball, or soccer. If you are over thirty-five years of age or are in poor health, check with your physician before starting any heavy exercise program.

If you have a difficult time getting out of the house each day to get your exercise, a stationary bicycle, or other exercise machine, is a good idea. Remember that almost anyone can walk for exercise from early childhood into advanced age.

Some Benefits of Regular Exercise

There are plenty of benefits to exercise. Regular exercise takes off unsightly bulges and, when coupled with the proper diet, helps shed excess pounds.

With sustained daily aerobic exercise the red blood cells begin to deliver additional oxygen to each body tissue cell. Through sustained exercise, the lungs gain the ability to be more efficient organs, able to deliver more vital oxygen from the air we breathe.

After a period of weeks or months of daily sustained exercise, the circulatory system produces an increased blood volume. This extra volume of blood provides additional hemoglobin that carries more oxygen and more red blood cells to the tissues. Additional blood plasma is produced as the entire blood volume increases. Some scientists have said that through proper exercise, blood volume can be increased by as much as one quart. The body ordinarily has about five quarts of blood, so this is an increase of 20 percent. With more red blood cells in the circulatory system, more oxygen is delivered to the entire body, and the body expels carbon dioxide and waste materials with more efficiency. The result is greater energy, less fatigue, and more vigorous health.[4]

Exercise also increases heart collateral circulation, meaning that the small blood vessels of the heart increase their ability to supply oxygen to the heart muscle. Kenneth E. Johnson, M.D., noted doctor of internal medicine and author, says: "In several well-documented cases, acute heart attacks and closure of one main heart artery did not result in sudden death. This protection occurred by virtue of the increased collateral circulation. Thus the heart muscle that would have been injured was not injured because of the collateral circulation.

"Exercise also helps prevent accidental blood clotting by lengthening clotting time. You'll have an easier time recovering from accidents and illness because of the additional oxygen carried in the blood."

As important as exercise is, the most important health issue is the type of fuel (food) you eat. The Miracle Diet program, made up basically of plants, starches, grains, vegetables, and fruits, is the basis for creating the *"Best Possible Health."*

Unfortunately, far too many people mistakenly believe that as long as they exercise often and vigorously they can continue eating red meat, fish, fowl, milk, cheese, butter, eggs, and vegetable fats. No one can stop the ongoing process of atherosclerosis with exercise, or medication, without changing his or her diet.[5] The Miracle program is the one that provides your body with the proper, healthful ratio of nutrients that promote health and prevent disease.

Supplement Exercise with Relaxation

In the complex world we live in today, we are all faced with tensions and stress which take their toll on our health.

Meditation and relaxation will help us cope with our problems and the day to day tension and stress in our lives.

If you want an on-the-spot remedy for stress, try relaxation or meditation techniques such as deep breathing (even for just a few seconds), progressive relaxation, mental focusing (using a single word or phrase), and muscle tensing and relaxing. All can bring about what is known as the "relaxation-response," the exact opposite of the "tension-stress" response. Blood pressure goes down, heart rate slows and the need for oxygen at the cell level is lessened. Respiration slows, stress hormones disappear from the bloodstream, and some scientists say that alpha and theta waves are produced in the brain, a sign of deep physiological and mental rest.[6-7]

Whatever you do, avoid addictive substances that are supposed to promote relaxation. Some chemical tranquilizers are addictive.

They soon become somewhat ineffective, and create negative effects in the body and mind. If you use tranquilizers or depend on pills for relief of tension and stress, stop! Replace them with *"The Miracle Diet"* it is a great help in relieving stress and tension. Stop the pills, become a Plantarian and exercise more.

For help, consult any of the many books on various relaxation techniques.[5-7] When practiced with *"The Miracle Diet"* program, relaxation techniques can help you enjoy the *"Best Possible Health"* physically, mentally, and spiritually.

Fifteen

Eating Out:
Restaurants, While Traveling
And With Friends

Okay, maybe you can follow *"The Miracle Diet"* at home, where you're in control of the kitchen. What happens when you're sitting in a restaurant?

Fast Food Options
No problem—as long as you tuck a few strategies under your belt!

Consider all the restaurants that feature salad bars. Even fast food outlets offer baked potatoes. Wendy's always has good plain baked potatoes for an inexpensive price. Fast food restaurants will prepare a good tomato and lettuce sandwich on a bun. Tell them if you want it with onions, pickles, and mustard. Wendy's has been very accommodating in making up these vegetable sandwiches; they are inexpensive. Wendy's also features a good salad bar. Sizzler has an excellent salad bar as well as baked potatoes, pasta, and other starch foods with little or no added fat. To have a healthy meal all you need to do is order a plain baked potato or potatoes (if you're really hungry), make up your own delicious salad out of plant food, and top it with vinegar or a fat-free dressing. Add plenty of bread, preferably whole wheat, but most any type bread will do, and you have a fast, tasty, filling, and healthy lunch or dinner.

Pizza
Call ahead and find a pizza parlor that uses whole wheat flour and a no-oil crust. Also ask if they use oil in their tomato sauce. Salt might be a problem if you are highly restricted, but otherwise you can manage fairly well.

You must be specific in your ordering of toppings. Order lots of oil-free tomato sauce as well as plenty of mushrooms, onions, tomatoes, and green peppers. Avoid cheese, pepperoni, and any other type of animal product.

Some make the pizza for you to bake at home, so you can control exactly what gets put on your pizza. Cook it in a non-stick pizza pan. This food is not the very best, but it can come fairly close to the program. Even Pizza Hut will custom-make you a vegetable pizza with lots of healthy toppings—but NO cheese.

Restaurant Eating

If a sit-down restaurant does not have a salad bar, you can usually order a la carte. Order a green salad with lots of added vegetables such as carrots, celery, onions, beets, green beans, broccoli, cauliflower, cabbage, and any other vegetables. Use a vinegar dressing, lemon juice, soy sauce or ask for a fat-free dressing. Then order a large plain baked potato or potatoes and plenty of whole wheat bread. Sourdough or rye is next best. But if the restaurant has only white bread or rolls—there is usually not much oil, salt, or sugar in bread compared to the total number of calories. And white bread is a great food compared to meat, fish, chicken, cheese, and eggs, all of which are laden with cholesterol and fat.

There are many other healthy choices on restaurant menus, such as cooked vegetables, boiled potatoes, plain rice, beans, corn, and peas. Order them with the least possible added oil and fat.

Cafeteria Choices

It's easy to find foods fairly compatible with The Miracle Diet program when you eat in a cafeteria. Most have a great variety of salads; look for those with the least amount of fats and dressings. Coleslaw and carrot salads usually have the lowest-oil dressings. Ask them to serve it dry or off the top.

Cafeterias usually have a good variety of cooked vegetables. Order those that usually contain the fewest fats. You can usually find good plain baked potatoes; if not, choose mashed potatoes. Plain rice or beans are other good choices in a cafeteria.

Fine Dining The Healthy Way

When you go out to an expensive restaurant you can still stay on the program. Order a plain baked potato or two (no butter, margarine or sour cream) as your entree accompanied by a delicious salad with extra raw vegetables and non-fat dressing. Order lots of good bread or rolls and eat plenty of cooked vegetables. Avoid fried foods.

Mexican Food Restaurants

Make some phone calls to find a Mexican food restaurant that does not use lard or vegetable fat in its beans. Many restaurants will gladly prepare your beans with no added fats if you ask in advance. Most chefs boil their beans the night before then refrigerate or freeze them. They add the lard, fats, and salt just before serving meals the next day. All you have to do is ask them to heat your beans without adding the lard, oils, and salt.

With these low-fat beans, the chef can make you a wonderful baked tostada on a corn and lime tortilla that has not been fried or a bean burrito with a soft whole wheat tortilla shell. Have the cook add all the extra tomatoes, lettuce, onions, and salsa you like. Be sure to tell the server you do not want any cheese, sour cream, avocado, guacamole, or olives added to your burrito.

Chinese Food Restaurants

Non-fat Chinese food is found in China, but not very often in American Chinese restaurants, but the basics for a healthy meal are still available.

Find a Chinese restaurant that serves whole-grain brown rice if possible, however, white rice is occasionally acceptable. Be sure to ask the server to have your vegetables cooked in light sauce that contains no oil or MSG (monosodium glutamate). Many Chinese restaurants now advertise no MSG in their food.

Good choices are vegetable chow mein or chop suey with plain rice. Ask them if their regular sauces or seasonings contain any oil. If so ask them to cook your vegetables in water. Learn to speak up and ask for healthy food. Some Chinese restaurants have a regular vegetable dish that is delicious and nourishing. Order lots of plain rice. Have them hold the oil. Tell them you are a Plantarian.

Japanese Food Restaurants

Japanese restaurants can serve you healthful meals if you will ask for no-oil or low-oil foods. Their basic foods, rice, and vegetables are part of The Miracle Diet program.

Let them know you are a Plantarian like many Orientals, and they will prize you as a customer.

Italian Food Restaurants

Call ahead and find an Italian restaurant that serves egg-free noodles. Also ask if they serve oil-free sauces, or will make up an oil-free sauce for you. Ask if they have oil-free soups, or will make up special soup for you that has no oil and is low on salt. Italian food can be very healthy if you leave off the meats, cheeses and fats.

Vegetarian or Health Food Restaurants

Many vegetarian or so-called "health food" restaurants are not always truly healthy. Some use lots of oil, eggs, and dairy products. Ask for oil-free rice, potatoes, beans, corn, and grains that have not been cooked with eggs or dairy products. Encourage them to provide for Plantarians and ask them to feature on their menu the *"Best Possible Health"* foods.

Just Speak Up

Do not hesitate to ask for what you want at a restaurant. Being a wise consumer can preserve your health, and even your life. Ask about the ingredients used in preparing restaurant dishes. Speak up for seconds if you are hungry. Request fat-free dressings and whole wheat breads. Ask for a little honey, jelly, or jam—a far better way to satisfy your taste for sweets than consuming rich sugar-and-fat-laden desserts.

For beverages you can order water, salt-free club soda, Perrier, or Sparkling water with a twist of lemon or lime, or unsweetened fruit juices.

When All Else Fails

On rare occasions you might find yourself in a situation where there are no healthy choices. Fill up on bread or ask if they have lettuce and tomatos—make a lettuce and tomato sandwich. Remember, this isn't your last meal. When you get home, there will be plenty of the proper foods to eat.

How to Cope When Traveling

What about traveling? That's when grocery stores solve the problem. Learn to stop at the store and buy your meals there. They even have disposable dishes and utensils if needed.

Let's start with breakfast. You could eat a dry cereal without sugar added, such as Grape-Nuts. Shredded Wheat is high in fiber with no added sugar or salt, and it's easy to eat while you drive, it's a good snack! If you must have milk, it should be fat-free soy milk or fat-free rice milk.

A good lunch is lettuce and tomato sandwiches on 100 percent whole wheat bread with carrots, onion, cucumbers, or other raw vegetables. Keep the best available 100 percent whole wheat bread in your vehicle when you are traveling. Another good bread is whole wheat pita (pocket) bread, which can be filled with cut-up vegetables. You can even make an entire meal out of good bread alone. Also try "Smart Beat" Fat-free Non-Dairy slices and you will have a "cheese" sandwich.

Motel Cooking

You can even carry along a small one or two-element hot plate, a few pots, and a small ice chest. In the evening, at the motel you can cook corn on the cob, frozen corn, peas, or any other frozen vegetables you like. You can boil potatoes in about 15 minutes. Carry good fruits, such as apples, bananas, oranges, and other fruits in season. A little frozen unsweetened fruit is good. This way of eating on the road costs a fraction of the cost of eating in restaurants, and the choices are unlimited at the grocery store.

"Eating Out" in the Supermarket

Many of the large supermarkets have good salad bars, as well as microwave ovens in the deli section. Buy yourself a sweet potato or white potato, one or two ears of corn, a carrot, and a tomato in the fresh vegetable section of the store. If you want a salad, pick that up at the salad bar. Take your potato and corn over to the deli and ask the clerk to cook your potato for six or seven minutes in the microwave oven on high setting, and your corn in the husk for four minutes. (Two ears take six minutes). Add some delicious rolls or bread. For dessert buy any fresh fruits. Some frozen yogurts are fat-free and cholesterol free. If you can tolerate dairy products they make a good dessert.

Air Travel—Special Meals

Those who travel by air have no excuse to stop eating properly. In the past few years, requests for vegetarian meals have been doubling each year on major air carriers. Good meals that are healthy can be obtained, but you must call twenty-four hours ahead of time to order a special meal. Request your travel agent to include your food preferences in your computerized reservation record. This will be on file, and every time you schedule a flight the correct meals will be automatically ordered.

Ask for the pure vegetarian, fat-free meals. If you are on a strict no-salt and/or low protein diet because of special health problems, you need to order a fruit plate. If you are on a small airline or a short flight that cannot accommodate your needs, carry your own food.

You "CAN" Take It With You

I usually carry some of my own healthy food such as a small container of cooked brown rice, a baked potato, some 100 percent whole wheat bread (a whole loaf on a long flight), and a few small baggies of raw vegetables and fruit.

Eating at Someone's Home

This can sometimes be a challenging experience. You have a choice: eat their food, and call it one of those seldom-do occasions, or eat light and pick and choose. In the long run, you will need to tell your friends you are following The Miracle Diet Program, that severely limits animal foods. Be courteous and not self-righteous. If your host is not acquainted with Plantarianism, politely explain that you've become convinced by medical breakthroughs that you want to severly limit your animal foods and fats.

If you are eating with close friends, it's simple. Just ask them to prepare a few extra vegetables and starches, especially staples like rice or potatoes without fats and little or no salt. Offer to bring something to add to the meal. Most of the group will enjoy your special dish and tell you how good it tastes.

Be a Good Example

Remember: your friends are also hearing in the news about cutting down on cholesterol and fat to prevent heart disease and most common cancers. Share *"The Miracle Diet"* books with your friends and let them know how to become even more attractive, lean and healthy. You can show them how to do it if they want to learn, but don't preach; just be a good example.

If you think the party or get-together will not feature enough of the proper food, or if you can't resist temptation, eat at home just before going out. It's easier to be strong when your stomach is full.

Sometimes when eating out or traveling you'll have to substitute a little. For example, you might get a little more salt and fat in restaurant vegetables and salads than what you want. If it isn't on a steady basis, you can still keep your fat intake fairly low. Don't resort to animal foods or fats on these special occasions because you might become addicted to them again.

Bend But Don't Break

Remember your goal is to become more attractive, lean and healthy, so don't be embarrassed about making special requests. You *won't* be the only one doing it. Many people are becoming more concerned about what they eat, and as restaurants get more requests they will add more healthy items to their menus.

A little inconvenience is a small price to pay for the benefits that will come to you. Remember, it's YOUR life and health that are at risk, and those are pretty high stakes!

Sixteen

Wise Consumers Know Their Numbers

Donuts may contain cholesterol and up to 80 percent highly saturated fat. Don't mistake donuts for a carbohydrate food. Don't be mislead by labels on ice cream, cheese, lunch meats, hot dogs, bacon and other foods that say 80 percent, 90 percent, 95 percent or even 97 percent fat-free. They may be going by total weight of the product, or some other method, instead of the percentage of calories (nutrients). The dairy industry has been telling us for many years that whole milk has only 3.5 percent fat. In reality, whole milk has nearly 50 percent of its calories as fat, mostly saturated fat, and it has a high cholesterol content. So-called low-fat milk (2 percent) is about 38 percent fat calories. Even skim milk contains from 5 to 10 mg. of cholesterol per eight-ounce glass.

Labels and The Law

The current laws concerning nutritional guidelines and labeling are very loose and conflicting, therefore food manufacturers can choose their interpretation of these laws. We need one hard and honest standardized method for measuring percentages of nutrients (fat, protein and carbohydrate) that will give a clear and concise picture to all consumers.

In spite of the present labeling dilemma, we can determine what percentage of fat we are consuming. To find out the true percentage of fat in any product, first multiply the number of grams of fat by 9 because there are 9 calories in every gram of fat. Then divide the number of fat calories by the total calories to determine the true percentage of fat calories per serving.

Example

Total calories per serving = 216

Grams of fat per serving = 12

12 x 9 = 108 fat calories, or 1/2 of the total calories

216 divided into 108 = .50 which means 50% fat calories

Many manufacturers now list total calories and fat calories as the first item. This is about the only meaningful information on these new labels. They list protein, carbohydrate and fat in grams. Fat is a more concentrated form of calories, containing 9 calories per gram compared to 4 calories per gram for carbohydrates and protein. This can be misleading because of the high calorie concentration in fat compared to protein and carbohydrate.

There's Lots of Confusion

Current 1994 food labeling requirements are very confusing. The percentages shown on the label do not reflect the actual percentage of nutrients in each serving of food.

The only information of any value in the 1994 labeling system is in the first section at the very top of the label. This shows **"Total Calories"** and **"Fat Calories,"** and with a little math you can quickly calculate the percentage of fat calories. For example, if total calories are 160 and fat calories are 80, you must divide 80 by 160 and you get .5 or 50% of calories from fat.

According to an article on present food labeling laws and nutrition, written in the Phoenix Gazette, March 20, 1995, nutritionists admitted that: "There's a great deal of confusion out there, especially when it comes to translating food labels into what to make for dinner." The present laws only require food companies to list the ingredients not even the amount of each ingredient. Contact your lawmakers in Washington, D.C. and demand a food label that is truly meaningful and understandable even for sixth grade school children. Also insist that the government begin implementing the **"New Four Food Groups"** in place of the present animal and milk food groups that are causing many unnecessary early deaths and diseases.

Food Labeling Should Be Clear and Concise

The true percentage of the total calories of each nutrient (fat, protein, carbohydrate) should be listed clearly on every food label.

The following example is for a 6 ounce helping of beef roast that is commonly consumed in the USA. Many people eat more than 6 oz. of meat for dinner. Remember 20 grams of fat should be our maximum fat intake per day if you want to be lean and healthy.

Example: Nutrition Facts Beef Chuck Roast	
Amount Per Serving . . . 6 oz.	
Calories 618	**Calories from Fat 444**
Total Fat 121 gm.	**72% Fat Calories**
Saturated Fat 49%*	
Polyunsaturated Fat 4%	
Monounsaturated Fat 47%	
Total Carbohydrate 0 gm.	**0% of calories**
Protein 47 gm.	**28% of calories**
Cholesterol 174 mg.	
Sodium 111 mg.	
Dietary Fiber 0 mg.	
*Human liver makes cholesterol out of saturated fat.	

All meat, chicken, fish, turkey, pork or lamb fresh, frozen or canned should be required by law to have the same food labeling.

By this clear and concise method all consumers would know exactly what they are eating and be informed, wise consumers.

Remember: 10% Fat or Less is Ideal

Each of us should be asking store managers to carry more products that are fat-free or low in fat. Write or call manufacturers and tell them you want healthier food products with little or no fat, no cholesterol and low sodium. Each of us can make a difference if we demand better labeling and healthier foods.

When you write or call your law makers to encourage them to adopt the **"New Four Food Groups"** also ask them to enact laws that make it mandatory to provide easy and concise labeling information as shown on page 114. You may copy sample label.

Be A Food Activist

Talk to elected school board members, school superintendents, principals and teachers about teaching up to date and better methods of nutritional principles. The percentage of nutrients (fat, protein and carbohydrate) in the foods we eat should be taught to all students. Charts listing the common foods should be on the walls of our classrooms so that students from first grade on up would learn to be informed consumers.[1]

School cafeteria items should have the percentages of nutritional ingredients listed clearly so students and teachers would know exactly what they are eating. The **"New Four Food Groups"** of WHOLE GRAINS, LEGUMES, VEGETABLES AND FRUIT should be taught to all students. This **"New Four Food Groups"** was introduced to the public early in 1991 by the Physicians Committee for Responsible Medicine, a nationwide group of physicians. For more information, write: Physicians Committee for Responsible Medicine, P.O. Box 6322, Washington, D.C., 20015, or telephone (202) 686-2210.

There is Light at the End of the Tunnel

The American Heart Association and American Cancer Society and other health organizations are calling for people to cut down on fat consumption. Most all health groups are now calling for Americans to cut fat consumption well below 30 percent. Dr. Art Ulene, M.D., noted NBC Today Show commentator, strongly advocates "cutting fat below 20 percent if you want to lose weight and be healthier too." Oprah Winfrey says: "20 grams of fat is ideal. That's about 10% fat calories. It is virtually impossible to cut your fat consumption if you do not know what percentage of fat is in each item of food you consume.

For the *"Best Possible Health,"* you should not eat more than 10% fat calories each day. On a 1500-calorie-per-day diet with 10 percent fat calories, 150 calories would come from fat. That equals about 16 1/2 grams of fat since there are 9 calories in every gram of

fat. The people in some counties of China eat less than 6% fat calories per day and seem to avoid many degenerative diseases.[2]

You need to realize that eating just one large, greasy doughnut
or Danish pastry containing 18 grams of fat could escalate your fat
intake for the day from 10 to 21 percent. This is more than twice the
fat intake for the *"Best Possible Health."* Don't be led down that
road into "Greasy City" by yielding to unbounded appetites!

Even the Industry is Responding

Good news is coming as we see huge food companies recognizing
the future markets for their products. For instance, in the Kraft
Foods quarterly financial report published July 1990, the lead story
was entitled, "Fat-free: The Next Generation," The article states:
"Every company has to ask itself, every day, 'What do our consumers
want?"

"At Kraft General Foods, we think we've found one answer: *fat-
free foods.*" Chairman and CEO, Michael A. Miles, said recently that
the company is "on the leading edge of one of the food industry's
biggest new product opportunities in years." Amazingly in 1994, over
1400 new fat-free or low-fat items came on the market.

Many other food companies are jumping on the "No-Fat, No-
Cholesterol Band Wagon." Health Valley Foods, based in California,
is a very progressive company. Their products are becoming available in supermarkets as well as health food stores. All supermarkets
should carry Fat-Free Soy Milk and Rice Milk. Fred Meyer supermarkets, a chain in six western states is a good example. They carry
a full line of healthy foods, grains, flours, beans, etc. More supermarkets would carry all types of natural whole grains, whole grain
flours, and other basic items that now are mostly found in health
food stores, IF there were more requests.

Seventeen

Shopping Hints and Suggestions

Visit a good supermarket or health food store for the following staples. You'll want to use many of these starches to replace animal foods and to supply the calories and energy you'll need every day. Also listed are other food items that fit into The Miracle Diet program, including seasonings and spices that enhance plant foods for enjoyable eating.

GRAIN PRODUCTS

WHOLE GRAINS
Wheat
Oats
Barley
Brown Rice
Corn
Rye
Millet
Bulgar Wheat

WHOLE-GRAIN FLOURS
Whole Wheat
Oat
Barley
Rice
Corn
Rye
Buckwheat
Whole wheat pastry

HOT WHOLE GRAIN CEREALS
Wheatena
Roman Meal
Zoom
Oatmeal
Oat bran
Cracked wheat
Barley
Seven-Grain

REFINED FLOURS
Gluten
White
White bread
White pastry
Semolina pasta

COLD WHOLE GRAIN CEREALS
Shredded Wheat
Grape Nuts
Nutra Grain
Kashi

WHOLE GRAIN PASTAS
Whole wheat and spinach
   spaghetti, macaroni,
Buckwheat Noodles
   lasagna
Corn pasta (not a wheat
   product)

There are many other
   acceptable cereals

**AVOID EGG NOODLES and
WHITE FLOUR PASTAS**

VEGETABLES

FRESH
Onions
Carrots
Cabbage (green and purple)
Scallions
Mushrooms
Celery
Bell Peppers
Tomatoes
Cucumbers
Zucchini
Broccoli
Cauliflower
Leeks
Iceberg lettuce, leaf lettuce
Radishes
Potatoes

FROZEN
Corn (is a grain, used as
   vegetable)
Asparagus
Peas (are legumes, used
   as vegetables)
Spinach
Hash brown potatoes
Okra
Cauliflower
Broccoli
Turnip greens
Collards
Green beans
Carrots
Onions

ROOT PLANTS

White potatoes
Yams
Sweet potatoes

CANNED (Caution: These
   are usually high in sodium)
Green beans
Stewed tomatoes
Beets

Rutabaga
Parsnips
Taro root
Water chestnuts
Jerusalem artichoke

Tomatoes
Tomato puree
Tomato juice
Corn
Peas
Beans (are legumes, used as
  vegetables)
Pimento
Green peppers
Jalapeno chili peppers

BEANS-LEGUMES

BEANS
Pinto
Navy
Red kidney
Black
Lima
Great northern
(Avoid soybeans; they are 40% fat)

PEAS
Split green
Whole green
Black-eyed

LENTILS
Brown
Green

("Beano" a gas prevention additive may be helpful)

FRUIT

FRESH
Oranges
Apples
Bananas
Peaches
Strawberries
Raspberries
Other fruits

FROZEN
Peaches
Strawberries
Raspberries
Blueberries

CANNED
Applesauce (unsweetened)
Apple juice
Pineapple (in own juice)
Pineapple juice
Pineapple juice concentrate
Orange juice concentrate

SPICES-HERBS

Allspice	Cilantro	Marjoram
Basil	Cinnamon	Mustard (dry)
Bay leaves	Cloves (ground)	Nutmeg
Black pepper	Coriander (ground)	Onion powder
Cardamom	Cumin	(salt-free)
Cayenne	Dill weed	Oregano
Celery seed	Garlic powder (salt-free)	Paprika
Chili powder	Ginger	Rosemary
Chives	Mace	Tarragon
		Tumeric

SEASONINGS AND CONDIMENTS

No-salt seasonings (Mrs. Dash)
Tomato ketchup
Salsa
Worcestershire sauce
Barbecue sauce
Mustard (regular or dijon)
Tabasco sauce
Vinegar
Soy sauce (low sodium)
Vanilla extract
Active dry yeast
Egg replacer (ENER-G)
Carob powder (unsweetened)

Swanson Chicken Broth (Fat
   Free, low sodium)
Baking powder
Beef broth (clear)
Baking soda
Corn starch
Salad dressings (Fat-free)
Honey
Pure maple syrup
Pure fruit jams and jellies
   (no added sugar)
Tapioca

Kitchen Equipment

To make cooking more fun and efficient, use the following equipment:

Stainless steel pots in graduated sizes
Non-stick bakeware (bread pans, cookie sheets, griddle,
   and frying pan)

Powerful blender or food processor
Hand mixer or electric hand mixer
Vegetable scrub brush
Colander
Garlic press
Hot-air corn popper
Pressure cooker
Crock-pot or slow cooker
Non-stick waffle iron
Juicer
Glass jars for sprouting seeds, beans, and grains
Double boiler (for cereals and sauces)
Wooden spoons
Grain grinding mill (for making your own flour and cereal)
Electric rice cooker (optional)
The Bread Machine (Welbilt, Regal, etc.) you'll love it.

What to Watch For—The Do's and Don'ts
Read All Labels

Remember that the food industry is trying to sell products, so you may get only elements of truth in their advertising. Check carefully for the oil and sugar content in processed commercial cereals, cookies, cakes, crackers, and breads. Buy food as natural and unrefined as possible.

Some examples of plain whole-grain cooking cereals are Wheatena, Zoom, oatmeal, oat bran, barley, and cornmeal. Most cold breakfast cereals are expensive, highly processed, and contain added sugars, salt, preservatives, and additives.

The federal government requires manufacturers to list the ingredients of any product in order of amount. The highest-volume ingredient is listed first, and the lowest-volume ingredient is listed last. Be constantly vigilant, because the food industry sometimes changes ingredients by adding sodium, syrups, sugars, oils, and fats to their products under various names. To avoid revealing high sugar content, many food companies list simple sugars such as corn syrup, sucrose, dextrose, fructose, or maltose instead of *sugar*.

Some products list separately the different kinds of fat—such as saturated, polyunsaturated, and monounsaturated. This is confusing because the label doesn't make much sense except for the first item at the top which lists total calories and calories from fat. Any product containing more than 10 percent fat will not produce the **"Best Possible Health."**

You may have heard that unsaturated fats are healthy, but saturated fats are not. Now for the facts: all added fats, animal or vegetable, are unhealthy if they exceed 10 percent. Many commercially manufactured bakery products, such as cakes, crackers, cookies, pies, doughnuts, bagels, rolls, and breads, are made with palm oil and/or coconut oil. Both of these oils are highly saturated vegetable oils, and the body produces cholesterol from saturated fat.

Caution: All vegetable oils contain too much saturated fat.

Example
Cottonseed Oil . . . . 27% Saturated Fat
Vegetable Shortening . . . . 26% Saturated Fat
Peanut Oil . . . . 18% Saturated Fat
Olive Oil . . . . 14% Saturated Fat
Corn Oil . . . . 13% Saturated Fat

It will amaze you how many calories we get from fats and oils in our food.
For example:
1 tablespoon of cooking oil or shortening = 14 grams, 125 calories.
1 cup of cooking oil or shortening = 218 grams, 1925 calories.
Butter and margarine contain nearly as many calories.

Many cake recipes call for 1 to 2 cups of fat. A slice of cake without fat may contain as little as 100 calories. The same slice of cake made with 1 cup of fat would contain 220 calories. The same cake made with 2 cups of fat would contain 340 calories per slice.

Many food products contain questionable additives. Sulfating agents as preservatives are added to many commercial dried foods and are used to keep salads looking fresh at restaurant salad bars. MSG (monosodium glutamate) is a sodium salt that is used as a flavor enhancer in many commercially packaged and canned foods. MSG can cause allergic reactions in many people, some of them serious. Americanized Chinese restaurants are big users of MSG. It would be wise to have your favorite restaurant hold the MSG and oil from your order.

Suggested Commercial Foods

Following are some packaged commercial foods that fit well into *"The Miracle Diet"* eating program. This is not an exhaustive list, but merely suggestions; read labels and find others on your own.

Frozen, Next Best to Fresh

Frozen foods are the number-one choice if fresh foods are not available or convenient as long as they do not contain additives. Frozen foods are nearly as healthy as fresh foods.

Avoid canned foods whenever possible. They are usually high in salt, sugar, and additives, and have fewer vitamins because of the heat processing. Finally, some of the metals in cans—such as lead, aluminum, and tin can be leached into the food.

Hot Cereals

As stated before, hot cooked cereals with the least processing possible are first choice. Try any of these:

Quaker Oats (regular or quick-cooking)   Wheatena
Oat Bran   Zoom
Seven-Grain Cereal   Roman Meal

The surest, safest, and least expensive way to enjoy cereals and flours is to grind your own. Buy an electric grain mill with a hand mill for emergency purposes.

Cold Cereals

The best choices are whole-grain cereals with no added fats or oils, little or no sugar, little or no salt, and few or no additives:

Health Valley Fat-free 10 Bran Cereal
Perky's Crispy Brown Rice
Shredded Wheat
Puffed Kashi, Seven Grains
Health Valley Organic Oat Bran Flakes
Grape-Nuts
Nature's Path Manna Oat Bran Flakes

Nutri-Grain (Wheat, Corn)

There are many others, but some brands are only found in health food stores.

Frozen Hash Brown Potatoes

Some frozen hash brown potatoes have no added fats, oils, or salt. Read labels carefully. Most of them have a little sugar (dextrose) and a preservative added.

Safeway Bel-Air Hash Browns (no preservatives)
Ore-Ida Hash Browns (preservatives-dextrose)
Mr. Dell's Hash Browns (no preservatives or additives)
Food Club Hash Browns (preservative-dextrose)

Popcorn

Air poppers and microwaves are good for popping corn. Use only unprocessed popcorn without any added ingredients. Any brand of popcorn can be used in an air popper. Popcorn with nothing added is a wonderful and filling complex carbohydrate starch. Plain kernel popcorn is inexpensive and can be found under a number of brand names in many types of stores. Spray your popped corn very lightly with water from a fine mist spray bottle as it comes out of the popper if you want a little salt to stick to it.

Crackers

Use wheat, rice, rye, and other seasoned whole-grain crackers with no added fats or oils. Read labels—some have added salt. Try these:

Westbrae Unsalted Brown Rice Wafers
Natural Ry-Krisp
Wasa Crispbread (Hearty Rye, Lite Rye)
Mini Crispys Rice Snacks
Weight Watchers Crispbread (Harvest Rice)
Nabisco's New, fat-free no cholesterol,
    low sodium cracker now available in supermarkets

Soups

Most canned soups are too high in fats, oils, and salt. If you wish to avoid milk and dairy products completely, the following dry packaged soups can be used:

Ramen (Whole Wheat, Onion, Curry, Miso, Carrot, Spinach, Seaweed, Mushroom)

Instant Miso Soup (Mellow White, Hearty Red)

Check your supermarket and health food store for acceptable soups. Some may have a high salt content, so read labels carefully. Try the following canned soups:

Hain's Split Pea Soup
Anderson's Split Pea Soup
Pritikin Lentil Soup
Health Valley Fat-free Soups

Pasta

Buy only egg-free pasta. Most pastas are made of flour and water with little salt and no added fats or oils. Use whole-grain (not refined flour) pastas. There are non-wheat pastas for people who are allergic to wheat. Many whole wheat and specialty pastas are found in the health food section in supermarkets or in health food stores.

Experiment with the many delicious varieties:

Westbrae Spaghetti Pasta (whole wheat, spinach)
Westbrae Lasagna Noodles (whole wheat, spinach)
Food for Health Spaghetti Pasta (whole wheat,
    spinach, artichoke, etc.)
Food for Health Macaroni, Rotini, Lasagna,
Udon (Japanese noodles, macaroni)
Japanese Buckwheat Pasta

Spaghetti Sauce

Most supermarket sauces contain large amounts of oil or fat and have a high salt content. Read labels carefully. For the best health, make your own sauce and freeze lots of it for future use. (See recipe for spaghetti sauce). You can find spaghetti sauce without oil in health food stores or in the health food sections at many supermarkets.

The following spaghetti sauces contain no meat or dairy products, no olive oil, and no other fats or oils:

Campbells Spaghetti Sauce (in a can)

Enrico's Spaghetti Sauce

Weight Watchers Spaghetti Sauce with mushrooms

Breads

There are many good 100 percent whole wheat, oat, seven-grain, wheat berry, and other whole-grain breads in supermarkets. Read labels carefully and choose those with the least oil, salt, and additives. They are not cheap, but buy the best. Orowheat makes many good quality breads. Local bakeries across the nation are making wonderful bread without any added fats.

Pita (pocket) breads generally have no added oils, fats, and sugars. They do have some salt; read labels carefully and know what you are eating. (Choose whole wheat over white).

If you are carefully avoiding fats in all of your other foods, good quality whole-grain breads that you buy in the supermarket are acceptable. If you are completely avoiding fats, salt, and sugars, stay with homemade breads or check breads found in health food stores. Most bread recipes can be modified to avoid oils, salt, and sugar to whatever extent you desire. Practice makes perfect.

Bread Machines

There are now bread machines on the market. All you have to do is place the ingredients in the machine, and about two to four hours later you have hot baked bread. You can even set the computer clock to have hot bread ready to eat at a specific serving time. Prices generally begin at $99.

If you are avoiding dairy products, the following breads are acceptable. Many are to be found only in health food stores. They have no added oil or dairy products, such as whey, and are low in sugar and salt. If you check labels carefully, you might also find some acceptable breads in your local grocery store.

Sprouted Seven-Grain Bread

Pritikin Bread (rye, whole wheat, multi-grain)

Sprouted Wheat with Raisin

Sprouted Rye Bread
Essene Bread
Bible Bread (regular and salt-free)
Mr. Pita

Baking Ingredients

All of these products are found in health food stores.

Featherweight Baking Powder
Rumford Baking Powder
ENER-G Egg Replacer (takes the place of eggs)

Many baking powders found in supermarkets contain aluminum.

Canned Tomatoes

There are a few tomato products you can buy in coated, lead-free cans if desired. Health Valley Foods is one brand available. Most canned tomato products will have high to fairly high salt content. Use salt-free if possible.

Real Frozen Desserts

If you are avoiding dairy products, even non-fat yogurt, use Fruit Sorbet, Fruit N' Juice Bars, and Dole Sun Tops. Another good choice is All-Natural Pops in various flavors made by Eskimo Pie Company. Other companies also make non-dairy frozen products to give you some acceptable treats from time to time.

Non-fat Soy Milks—Rice Milks

They taste better than cow's milk and are sweeter and can be stored, before opening, for long periods of time.

Use these milks in place of non-fat cow milk products in cooking and on cereals. Fat-free soy milk and fat-free rice milk are available in health food stores and some supermarkets. If you can't find fat-free soy milk or fat-free rice milk, use 1% and dilute. Mix three parts water to one part soy milk.

Health Valley Fat-Free Soy Moo
Westsoy Non-fat Soy Milk by Westbrae
Edensoy 1% Soy Milk

Pacific Rice Milk Fat-Free
Imagine Foods 1% Rice Dream Milk

Seasoning Mixes-Salt-Free
Many combinations of vegetables and spices are made with no added salt. Two regular brands are:
Mrs. Dash (Original Blend, Extra Spicy,
    No Garlic-Low Pepper, Extra Fine Grind)
Vegit All-Purpose Seasoning

Salsas
Salsa contains only vegetable ingredients, and no oils. There are preservatives in some, and many have salt, sugar, or both-so read labels carefully. Better yet, make your own! (See salsa recipe.)

Pace Picante Sauce	Territorial House
Old El Paso Salsa	La Victoria

Soy Sauces
Soy sauces contain no MSG (monosodium glutamate). Use somewhat sparingly as they are all high in sodium, though some are salt-reduced:
San-J Tamari Wheat-Free Soy Sauce
Westbrae Mild Soy Sauce
Kikkoman Lite Soy Sauce

Other Sauces with No Oil
A-1 Steak Sauce
Bullseye Barbecue Sauce
K.C. Masterpiece Barbecue Sauce
Tabasco Sauce
Hunt's Thick and Rich Barbecue Sauce
Heinz Worcestershire Sauce
French's Worcestershire Sauce
Cajun Sunshine

Some are much higher in salt and in sugar than others. Hunt's makes a no-salt ketchup. Heinz makes a "lite" ketchup with reduced salt and sugar. Westbrae makes an unsweetened ketchup.

No-Fat Canned Bean Products

Many supermarkets now stock all types of canned beans without added fat and salt. Check the labels. Health Valley makes a fat-free chili with black beans. There are several brands of Fat-free refried beans.

> Janet Lee Great Northern Beans
> Kuner's Black-eyed Peas
> Kuner's Great Northern Beans
> Old El Paso Fat-free Refried Beans
> Shur-Fine Red Kidney Beans
> Old El Paso Pinto Beans
> Rosarita No Fat Refried Beans

Now there is **"BEANO THE GAS PREVENTER"**: "A scientific breakthrough!" According to their advertising this product "prevents the gas from beans and cabbage, peas, broccoli, eggplant and many others." All the people I know who have tried this product really like it. I have tried it too and it works.

Jams, Jellies and Syrups

Use a limited amount of natural-fruit jams, jellies, and syrups that have no added sugar, corn syrup, or other sugars, and very few, if any, preservatives. You can use pure honey or maple syrup, but only with caution and in limited amounts.

> Smucker's Simply Fruit (red raspberry, strawberry, blueberry, boysenberry, apricot, blackberry, orange marmalade)
> North Farm Spreadable Fruit (apricot, strawberry, raspberry)
> Sorrell Ridge 100% Fruit (orange marmalade, etc.)
> Welch's Totally Fruit (boysenberry, apricot, blueberry, strawberry, red raspberry, blackberry, orange marmalade)

Salad Dressings

Salad dressings should be free of oil and should have little salt. Watch the salt content carefully; it might be high, even in the no-oil brands.

> Kraft Miracle Whip FREE
> Fat-free and Cholesterol Free

Kraft FREE Mayonnaise Dressing
    Fat-free and Cholesterol Free
Pritikin Oil Free (Italian, French, Vinaigrette, Russian)
Kraft Fat-Free (Italian, French, Thousand Island,
    Ranch, Catalina)
Seven Seas Fat-Free (Italian, Ranch, Red Wine)
Hidden Valley Fat-free Ranch and others
Regina Red Wine Vinegar with garlic flavor

Cookies, Cakes, Muffins

New fat-free, cholesterol-free baked items are coming on the market. Be sure to read all labels.

Health Valley Cookies (apricot, raisin oatmeal,
    apple spice, date, Hawaiian fruit, raspberry)
Health Valley Muffins (blueberry, apple spice, banana,
    raisin spice)
Entenmann's fat-free and cholesterol-free
    baked goods (golden cake, chocolate loaf cake,
    oatmeal raisin cookies)
Nabisco Snackwell's Fat-free (several kinds)
Nabisco Fat-free Fig Newtons (raspberry, strawberry, etc.)

No Fat Oat Fruit Bars

Many new delicious fruit bars, candies and other heathy snack items are coming on the market. Look for Health Valley, No Fat, or No Fat Added Oat Bran Fruit Bars. These take the place of rich, fat, sugar laden, high calorie candy bars.

Tortilla Corn Chips

NEW! Guiltless Gourmet No Oil Tortilla Corn Chips. No saturated fat, no cholesterol. Baked not fried, salted or no salt. Now in Health food stores and Supermarkets. Make your own. (See recipe)

Frito-Lay makes: Baked Tostitos with no added fat
Fat-free Baked Rold Gold Pretzels
Louise's Fat-free Potato Chips

Eighteen

Two Weeks of Easy Menus

If you don't like to spend much time cooking, *"The Miracle Diet"* program is the answer!

Follow this outline of which foods you need to have on hand to start. Adjust according to family size. You may already have some of these staples, in your cupboards.

Shopping List

10-20 lbs. whole-grain wheat
5-10 lbs. whole wheat flour
5-10 lbs brown rice
10 lbs. potatoes
10 lbs. dry corn
5 lbs. cornmeal
4 pkgs. frozen green vegetables
2 pkgs. frozen corn
Various fresh or frozen fruits
   and vegetables
2 cans tomatoes
2 cans tomato juice
Cornstarch or arrowroot
Vinegar (white, cider, wine)
Dried fruits (such as raisins)
2 lbs. barley
Honey
Tomato ketchup (low-sodium)
Salad dressings (oil-free, low-sodium)

Baking soda (without MSG)
Soy milk (Fat Free)
Whole wheat pita bread
100 percent whole wheat bread
5 lbs. popcorn
Pasta sauce (oil-free, low-sodium)
10 lbs. pinto beans
5 lbs. navy beans
5 lbs. lima beans
5 lbs. carrots
10 lbs. onions
1 42-oz. box regular oatmeal
2 16-oz. boxes oat bran (cereal)
2 20-oz. boxes Wheatena
   (cereal)
Pure fruit jams and jellies
   (with no sugar added)
Fat-free, low-salt Mexican salsa
Soy sauce (low-sodium)

2 bunches celery

Baking powder (without aluminum)

Non-animal egg replacer (ENER-G)

36-pack corn and lime only tortillas

Lemon juice (bottled)

Maple syrup (pure)

5 lbs or more pastas (whole wheat and vegetable)

Beverages

Postum, Pero, or other cereal drink

Soda water or seltzer Water (sodium-free, add fruit juices for variety)

Herbs and Seasonings

Salt-free mixed seasoning (i.e. Mrs. Dash)

Garlic powder

Cayenne pepper

Nutmeg

Dill weed

Onion powder

Cinnamon

Black pepper

Oregano

Parsley flakes

Simple Eating the First Two Weeks

During the first two weeks on this program your body will begin to heal itself; at the same time, you'll be getting used to new and exciting tastes. You will soon learn to prefer this simple and inexpensive way to eat. Your energy level should increase and you'll be amazed by how much better you'll feel.

Typical Meals the First Two Weeks

Recipes for some of these foods are detailed in a later chapter.

WEEK ONE
Day One

Breakfast:

Wheatena cereal, double helping; follow package instructions. Use fat-free soy milk or fat free rice milk. Eat an orange or other fruit if you are still hungry.

Lunch:

Tomato Burger (recipe on page 176) Serve with baked chips and a variety of cut-up raw vegetables, such as broccoli, cauliflower, onion, celery, carrots, or radishes. Eat an apple, applesauce, or other fruit for dessert.

Dinner:

One, two, or more baked potatoes; a fresh or frozen green vegetable; green salad; whole wheat bread; soda water optional (plain or mixed with fruit juice). Banana or any fruit of choice for dessert. Keep small bags of cut up bananas in the freezer ready to create a soft ice cream-like dessert or snack any time: place equal amounts of frozen bananas and any sugar-free frozen fruit (i.e. raspberries, strawberries, peaches) in a blender. Blend, with a little water, fat-free rice or soy milk if necessary. This treat is all complex carbohydrates.

To prepare potatoes, microwave one for about 6 minutes, microwave two for 9-10 minutes, or bake six or more in the oven for an hour at 400°; store unused potatoes in the refrigerator for future use.

Snacks:

Snack on air-popped popcorn; home-baked corn tortilla chips (to make chips, cut corn tortillas in eighths, bake for 30 min. in a 350° preheated oven) or other fat-free, low-sodium foods. Aim for complex carbohydrates. You can eat these throughout the day-you'll never be hungry! *Guiltless Gourmet* is a brand name found in health food stores. They produce a no oil, baked tortilla chip. Baked Tostitos by Frito-Lay are also very tasty.

Day Two

Breakfast:

Oatmeal, double portion; follow instructions on box. Eat an orange or other fruit if desired. (If your triglyceride level is over 200, limit your fruits to one a day and cut out other simple sugars.

Lunch:

Vegetable soup or stew (eat plenty!), whole wheat bread, and an apple.

Dinner:

Brown rice (heat up 1 or 2 cups precooked and eat it plain or with a little black pepper); fresh or frozen peas; summer squash; raw vegetable salad (use six or more vegetables with an oil-free, low-sodium dressing); whole wheat bread with fruit jam; sliced bananas with applesauce and cinnamon for dessert. Angel food cake is acceptable as an occasional treat.

Day Three

Breakfast:

Two quarts mixed-grain cereal (1 cup of dry mix makes one quart of cereal); stir occasionally and thin by adding water while cooking. Prepare without adding milk or sugar. Cooking time is 15 minutes or more.

Lunch:

Whole wheat pita (pocket) bread filled with a variety of cut-up raw vegetables; add pre-cooked rice or beans for variety. Eat two or three pitas if you are hungry; dessert, fruit of your choice.

Dinner:

Pinto beans; yellow or green cooked vegetable; a variety of raw vegetables; and applesauce or fruit for dessert. Always keep pre-cooked pinto beans without added fat or salt in the refrigerator and freezer so you can prepare a fast, easy meal on a moment's notice. Add salt at table if necessary.

Day Four

Breakfast:

Shredded Wheat cereal with fat-free soy or rice milk, apple juice; fruit if desired.

Lunch:

Vegetable stew; whole wheat bread or pita bread; fruit for dessert if desired, or Snack Well brand fat-free cookies.

Dinner:

One or two baked potatoes (white or sweet), plain or with fat-free salad dressing as a topping; two ears of cooked corn; green cooked vegetable; raw vegetables or salad. For dessert, cold cooked brown rice with banana and a little cinnamon. To prepare ears of corn in the microwave, shuck the corn and place it in a plastic bag; cook one ear on high setting for about four minutes, two ears for six minutes.

Day Five

Breakfast:

Hash-browned potatoes, fresh or frozen. If you buy frozen, be sure there are no added fats or preservatives. Cook in a non-stick pan or griddle over medium-high heat for about 15 min. on one side and 10 min. on the other. Diced onion adds flavor. Add ketchup for more flavor.

Lunch:

Bean Burger (recipe on page 176); salad made of five or six raw vegetables; Serve with baked chips.

Dinner:

Two or three ears of corn; frozen green vegetable; mixed vegetable salad with non-fat dressing. Applesauce for dessert.

Day Six

Breakfast:

Grape Nuts with fat-free soy or rice milk, apple juice, orange, banana, or other fruit.

Lunch:

Lettuce, tomato, onion, and/or cucumber sandwich on whole wheat bread; one baked potato; a variety of raw vegetables.

Dinner:

Precooked pinto beans; frozen spinach or other green vegetable; whole-grain bread; raw vegetable salad with fat-free dressing; apple or other fruit for dessert. NOTE: Eat beans, peas, or lentils only every other day or no more than one cup each day otherwise you may get too much protein. A variety of canned beans are now available with no added fat. You can also buy salt-free canned beans.

Day Seven

Breakfast:

Seven-grain cooked cereal, preferably without milk to get the full flavor of the grains; half a grapefruit. Seven-grain cereal can be found in health food stores, or make up your own cereal by combining several grains.

Lunch:

Boca Burger (fat-free) recipe on page 177; soda water or seltzer water (optional) with or without added natural fruit juice. Serve with Baked Tostitos.

Dinner:

Mashed potatoes, whipped with Mrs. Dash, pepper, and fat-free soy milk or fat-free rice milk; mixed vegetable salad with oil-free, low-sodium dressing; yellow or green cooked vegetable. Strawberries (without added sugar) and some fat-free cookies for dessert. There are more fat-free cookies coming on the market.

WEEK TWO

Use any combination of foods or menus from week one, as long as you stay with plant food using the five basic starches (beans, potatoes, brown rice, corn, and grains) as your major source of calories. Vegetables and fruits should make up the balance of your calories. These simple foods take practically no preparation if you fill your refrigerator with precooked starches (such as beans, brown rice, winter squash and oven-baked potatoes), bagged cut raw vegetables, and fruit. Plant foods do not spoil as quickly as animal foods, so you can cook a large amount of food at one time and keep it in the refrigerator for up to two weeks without spoilage. Most plant foods freeze well, too.

Other Easy Meal Suggestions:

Bean Tostados made with steamed corn tortillas, topped with fat-free refried beans, chopped lettuce, tomatoes, onions (optional), fat-free salsa.

Veggie soft taco, made with fat-free refried beans, (you can find these canned beans in your supermarket). Add lettuce, tomatoes, onions and salsa.

Veggie pizza with lots of veggies, lots of sauce (fat-free of course), no cheese. See bread section for pizza crust.

Go to Subway, get a veggie sandwich on wheat bread, with lots of veggies, use mustard, no cheese, no mayo, no olives.

NOTE: 100% whole wheat bread is the staff of life and can be eaten with every meal and between meals as snacks. A little jam preferably 100% fruit jams, no added sugar or honey can make great snacks and desserts. One hundred years ago, or more, our ancestors ate over a pound of 100% whole grain bread per person per day.

Bread machines sell for as low as $99.00. They make great whole grain bread without much work and require no previous experience. That makes it easy to have plenty of nutritious no-fat-added, 100% whole wheat bread at every meal. (See bread recipe.)

Note: For maximum weight loss do not eat food containing highly milled (like white) flour.

Nineteen

7 Days of Easy Menus and Recipes
for People Who Like to Cook

If you enjoy cooking, you'll find the following week of menus to be satisfying, delicious, and good for you! Don't get bogged down following the menus exactly: pick and choose, and create your own. And don't limit yourself to the recipes listed here; some other cookbooks feature recipes that follow The Miracle Diet program. *"The Miracle Diet Cookbook,"* companion to this information book, features nearly 400 more delicious recipes.

Note that many of the following recipes call for precooked rice or beans. Cook these up in quantity, and freeze them in conveniently sized packages. You'll have delicious gourmet meals in minutes as a result!

Be sure to look for *The Miracle Diet Cookbook*
Fat-Free • Cholesterol Free • High Fiber
now available at your favorite bookstore or by calling 1-800-922-9681

Day One
Breakfast:
HOT MIXED CEREAL
4 cups water
1 cup dry mixed cereals (equal parts Wheatena, oat bran, regular oats-keep a large covered container of pre-mixed dry cereal on hand)
Raisins or other fruit (optional)
(Each cup of dry cereal makes about 1 quart of cooked cereal.)
Bring the water to a boil in a saucepan. Add the pre-mixed cereal, stir, reduce heat to medium-low, and stir occasionally. For smoother cereal, cook longer; turn to low heat if you want to cook longer than 15 minutes. Add water to thin mixture if needed. Add fruit if desired.

Serves: 1
Preparation Time: 2 minutes
Cooking Time: 10-20 minutes

Lunch:
LETTUCE, TOMATO, ONION, AND CUCUMBER SANDWICH

2 slices whole wheat bread   lettuce leaves

1 sliced tomato   sliced cucumbers

1 mild onion, sliced   dressing (oil-free and low-sodium)

black pepper, Mrs. Dash

Toast bread if desired; spread dressing on bread. Layer tomatoes, onion, and cucumbers on one slice, cover with lettuce. Spice with a little Dijon mustard if desired. Serve with baked chips. Garnish with fresh radishes, cauliflower, and celery.

Dinner:
FANTASTIC SPAGHETTI SAUCE

2 cans (28-oz.) tomatoes, slightly chopped

2 cans (29-oz.) tomato sauce

3 cups chopped onion

2 cups chopped bell pepper

5 or 6 cups sliced mushrooms

1 tablespoon garlic, minced

2 tablespoons wine vinegar

2 tablespoons basil

2 teaspoons Mrs. Dash mixed spices and herbs

Combine all ingredients, except basil, in a large saucepan or skillet. Simmer about 1 hour; add basil and simmer 30 minutes longer. You can make the sauce early in the day and reheat just before serving. About 15 minutes before serving, drop 1 pound of egg-free whole wheat or spinach spaghetti into 4 quarts boiling water and cook until tender, or about 10 minutes. Serve with sauce. Freeze leftover sauce for future use.

    Servings: 10-12

    Preparation Time: 15 minutes

    Cooking Time: 1 1/2 hours

Salad:

Serve a mixed vegetable salad of broccoli, cauliflower, green onions, carrots, purple cabbage, and lettuce; garnish with fat-free dressing.

Dessert:

SPICE CAKE

1/2 cup brown sugar	1/2 teaspoon nutmeg
1 cup whole wheat flour	1/2 cup applesauce
1 cup white flour	1 cup raisins
1/4 teaspoon soda	1/2 cup chopped dates (optional)
3 teaspoon baking powder	1 cup nonfat soy milk
1 teaspoon cinnamon	3 teaspoons egg replacer
1/4 teaspoon cloves	ENER-G or 2 egg whites

Mix all ingredients. Bake in 8"x8" non-stick pan at 350° for 30 to 45 minutes, or until toothpick comes out clean. (Vanilla sauce, recipe below)

VANILLA SAUCE

2 cups nonfat soy milk	1/2 cup brown sugar
3 tablespoons cornstarch	1 teaspoon vanilla

Cook together until thick. Remove and add 1 teaspoon vanilla. Serve hot over spice cake.

> Servings: 12-16
> Preparation Time: 30 minutes
> Cooking Time: 30-45 minutes

Day Two

Breakfast:

FROZEN HASH-BROWN POTATOES

1 package frozen hash-brown potatoes (choose a brand with no added oil)
1/2 cup chopped onion
1/8 teaspoon Mrs. Dash
pepper to taste

Cook in a nonstick skillet over medium heat for 15 minutes; turn and cook for 10 minutes on other side, until browned. Garnish with ketchup or other sauce (no-oil).

> Servings: 1 (eat all you want)
> Preparation Time: 1 minute
> Cooking Time: 25 minutes

Lunch:

TOMATO BURGER

(Recipe on page 176.) Serve with baked chips (California Bakes—Hot and Smoky Chipotle) These are tasty!

Dinner:

TAMALE PIE CASSEROLE

4 cups cooked mashed pinto beans
  (you may use No Fat Refried canned beans)
2 chopped onions
2 teaspoons chili powder
1/2 cup tomato sauce
1 1/2 cups frozen or canned corn
8-12 oz. can chopped green chiles
2 cups cornmeal
3 cups water

Cook onions in 1/2 cup water for 10 minutes. Add chopped green chiles, corn, tomato sauce and 1 teaspoon of the chili powder. Cook 5 minutes, add beans and cook another 10 minutes over low heat. Remove from heat.

Combine cornmeal with balance of water and the rest of the chili powder in a saucepan and cook over medium heat until mixture thickens, stirring constantly to keep cornmeal from lumping.

Using a 9"x13" non-stick pan, spread half of the cornmeal mixture over the bottom. Pour the bean mixture over this and spread it out. Put the remaining cornmeal mixture over the top and bake at 350° for 45 minutes, or until it bubbles.

  Servings: 8
  Preparation Time: 45 minutes
  Cooking Time: 45 minutes

Vegetable:
COOKED BROCCOLI, FRESH OR FROZEN
Place 1/4 inch of water in a medium saucepan; add frozen broccoli, bring to a boil, and cook 10 minutes, or until tender. Cook fresh broccoli about 20 minutes.

Salad:
COLESLAW
4 cups shredded cabbage
1 medium carrot, shredded
1 onion, finely chopped
2 teaspoons sugar
Dash of salt
1/2 cup fat-free soy milk, or Kraft NO-FAT Miracle Whip
Dash of paprika
Combine all ingredients but paprika; sprinkle paprika on top.
> Servings: 6
> Preparation Time: 20 minutes
> Cooking Time: none

Dessert:
BAKED FRUIT SALAD SUPREME
1 16-oz. can pineapple chunks (in own juice, drained with juice reserved)
1 tablespoon tapioca
1 fresh apple, diced
1 orange, peeled and diced
4 tablespoons frozen pineapple juice concentrate
2 egg whites
1/8 teaspoon cream of tartar
1/2 teaspoon vanilla
2 teaspoons sugar (optional)
Bring reserved pineapple juice and tapioca to a boil until thickened. Combine the apple, pineapple, orange, and frozen pineapple juice concentrate. Mix well to coat fruits with the thickened juice. Spoon fruit into 4 individual souffle baking dishes. Beat egg whites until soft peaks form. Add the cream of tartar and sugar and continue beating until stiff peaks form. Add vanilla. Swirl the egg whites to top of the fruit salad, heaping it thick and spreading it to edges of dishes. Place in pre-heated 450° oven for 4 to 5 minutes until meringue is lightly browned.
> Servings: 4
> Preparation Time: 20 minutes
> Cooking Time: 10 minutes

Day Three

Breakfast:
APPLE PIE WAFFLES OR PANCAKES

1 3/4 cups fine whole wheat flour

1 teaspoon honey

1/2 cup wheat bran

1 cup non-fat soy milk

2 teaspoons dry yeast

1/2 teaspoon salt , optional

1 teaspoon apple pie spice

2 apples, grated

3 tablespoons applesauce

3/4 cup warm water

2 teaspoons egg replacer mixed with 4 tablespoon water or 2 egg whites

Mix flour, bran, apple pie spice, and salt (optional); set aside. Combine yeast, water, and honey, and let rest 5 minutes while grating peeled apples. Add the soy milk, applesauce, egg replacer, or egg whites and grated apple to the yeast mixture. Mix well and combine with the dry ingredients. Cover and let rest for 15 minutes. Pour about 1 cup of batter into a hot waffle iron and cook for 7-8 minutes, or until the lid lifts easily.

Pancakes: Ladle batter onto a medium-hot, nonstick griddle and flatten cakes so the center will cook. Cook about 10 minutes on first side, about 6-8 minutes on the other. Don't turn until bubbles form on top. These cakes are thicker than regular pancakes and take longer to cook. Note: Lightly oil a nonstick waffle iron before heating to prevent sticking. To keep warm before serving, place cooked waffles in a warm oven on a bare oven rack.

Servings: makes 14 pancakes or 4 waffles

Preparation Time: 30 minutes

Cooking Time: 20 minutes

Resting Time: 15 minutes

Lunch:
PITA BREAD STUFFED WITH BROWN RICE & VEGGIES

1 or 2 pieces pita bread

1 cup precooked brown rice

Suggested vegetables:

    Cucumber, sliced

    Tomato, chopped

    Carrot, grated

    Yellow onion, chopped

    Celery, chopped

Mexican salsa, optional (oil-

    free, low-sodium)

Broccoli, chopped

Green pepper, chopped

Lettuce leaves

Green onion, chopped

Cauliflower, chopped

Fill the pita with all or any combination of vegetables; add salsa if desired.

    Servings: 1

    Preparation Time: 10 minutes

    Cooking Time: none

Dinner:
TOASTED RICE PILAF

To toast rice, spread a cup or two of brown rice in a shallow baking sheet, one layer deep. Bake at 325° to 425° F. for 10-25 minutes, stirring occasionally. Let rice cool, store in canister or jar and cook just as you would plain rice.

3 cups cooked brown rice (made from toasted rice)

2 cups sliced mushrooms

2 1/2 cups beef broth (defatted)

4 teaspoons dehydrated onion flakes

4 teaspoons minced parsley

Combine ingredients in casserole, mix well, and bake at 375° F. for 25-35 minutes, until piping hot.

    Servings: 4

    Preparation Time: 30 minutes

    Cooking Time: 25-35 minutes

Vegetable:
COOKED CABBAGE
Place 1/2 inch of water in saucepan; add 1/2 cut up cabbage; cook over medium-high heat until cabbage is barely tender (about 5 minutes). Do not overcook; cabbage should be crunchy.

Salad:
CARROT-RAISIN SALAD
4 carrots, grated/shredded
1/4 cup raisins
4 oz. crushed pineapple with juice (1/2 small can)
Blend all ingredients well. To blend flavors better, refrigerate a few hours before serving.

Servings: 4
Preparation Time: 5-10 minutes

Dessert:
APPLE CRISP
2 cans sliced apples (water-packed)   1/4 cup honey
1 cup chopped dates   1 cup pineapple juice
Apple pie spice to taste   (unsweetened)
1 tablespoon lemon juice   1 teaspoon cinnamon
1/2 cup wheat flakes, quick oats,   1 1/2 cups whole wheat flour
  or Grape-Nuts   1/2 cup frozen apple juice
                                         concentrate (undiluted)

Fill an 8" by 8" nonstick pan with the apple slices. Sprinkle with chopped dates. Add pineapple juice. Sprinkle with apple pie spice to taste (approximately 1-2 tablespoons). Mix flour and wheat flakes, quick oats, or Grape-Nuts; if you use Grape-Nuts, crush with a rolling pin. Add apple juice a little at a time and toss with a fork. Sprinkle mixture over apples. Bake in 350° oven for 15-30 minutes.

Serves: 6
Preparation Time: 15 minutes
Cooking Time: 15-30 minutes

Day Four

Breakfast:

QUICK OATMEAL

1/2 cup quick-cooking oatmeal; 1 cup water, or
1 cup quick-cooking oatmeal; 2 cups water
Place water in pot. Add oats, bring water to a boil, and stir. Boil for 1
minute, stirring occasionally. Cover pot, turn off heat, and remove from
burner. Wait 4 to 5 minutes, stir, and serve. Eat plain, or with a little cinnamon or nutmeg. For variety, add raisins or other dry fruits during or after
cooking.

 Servings: 1
 Preparation Time: 2 minutes
 Cooking Time: 4 minutes

Lunch:

BAKED POTATO

Scrub potato; bake in microwave oven for 6 minutes. Sprinkle with pepper
and Mrs. Dash. Serve warm or cold with whole wheat bread and a variety of
cut vegetables.

 Servings: 1
 Preparation Time: 2 minutes
 Cooking Time: 6 minutes

Dinner:

RICE CASSEROLE

1 cup cooked brown rice	1 cup sliced mushrooms
1/2 cup non-fat soy milk	2 cups canned tomatoes, diced
Whole wheat bread crumbs	1 cup chopped green pepper
1/2 cup chopped onion	1/2 teaspoon Mrs. Dash
1/4 teaspoon black pepper	Dash of paprika

Mix vegetables, soy milk, and seasonings. Mix with rice and put in a non-
stick covered casserole dish, or spray lightly with nonstick coating spray.
Cover with whole wheat bread crumbs. Bake in 350° oven about 45 minutes.
To cook brown rice: Place 2 1/2 cups water in a 3-quart saucepan. Bring to a
boil. Add 1 cup rice and cover pan. Turn to low heat and steam for 45 minutes or until water evaporates.

 Servings: 6
 Preparation Time: 15 minutes
 Cooking Time: 45 minutes

Vegetable:
GLAZED CARROTS
8 large carrots, thinly sliced
1/4 cup undiluted frozen apple juice, thawed
1 tablespoon grated orange rind
1 teaspoon cornstarch
1/8 teaspoon ground cloves
Steam carrots over boiling water for 15 minutes, or until tender. Combine apple juice, orange rind, cornstarch, and cloves in a saucepan. Mix until smooth, then cook and stir constantly until mixture has thickened and cleared. Add the cooked carrots to the sauce. Serve hot.

    Servings: 8

Dessert:
RASPBERRY FROZEN DESSERT
1 1/2 cups canned unsweetened crushed pineapple with juice
3 frozen bananas
3 cups frozen raspberries (1 16-oz. bag, low sugar)
To freeze bananas, peel, cut up, and freeze in a plastic bag for at least 12 hours. Place the pineapple with juice and bananas in the blender. Add the frozen raspberries a little at a time, blending well. Place 1/2 cup of mixture into each of 8 dessert dishes and freeze for 15-30 minutes. If ingredients are frozen for a longer period of time, remove from freezer a short while before serving.

    Servings: 8
    Preparation Time: 10 minutes
    Cooking Time: none (requires
      15-30 minutes freezing time)

Day Five

Breakfast:

COLD RICE-CEREAL-FRUIT COMBO

2/3 cup cooked rice

Add any fat-free, sugar free cold cereals. Top with any fruit; raisins, bananas, berries, etc. Add a dash of cinnamon.

For liquid use apple juice, or non-fat soy or rice milk.

> Servings: 1
> Preparation Time: 2 minutes
> Cooking Time: none

Lunch:

GRILLED CHEESE SANDWICH
(Recipe on page 177.)

POTATO SALAD

6 cups diced cooked potatoes	1 cup Kraft Fat-free
1-2 medium onions, chopped	Mayonnaise or Miracle Whip
1 tablespoon mustard	3/4 cup sweet relish
1/2 cup diced celery	salt and pepper to taste

Combine all ingredients; mix well.

Whole-grain bread, raw vegetables, and/or non-fat corn tortilla chips go well with potato salad.

Servings: 6-8

Preparation Time: 20 minutes

Cooking Time: none

Dinner:
VEGETABLE CHOP SUEY
1/4 cup water
2 onions
2 cloves garlic, crushed
1 stalk celery, sliced
1/4 pound broccoli, sliced
1 cup snow peas
1 cup bean sprouts
1/4 pound mushrooms, sliced
1/2 cup green onions, sliced in one-inch pieces
3 or 4 tablespoons cornstarch
3 cups water
3 tablespoons low sodium soy sauce

Place 1/4 cup water into large pot or wok; add crushed garlic, and heat water to boiling. Add onions, celery, mushrooms, and broccoli. Saute about 10 minutes and add the water, soy sauce, green onions, snow peas, and bean sprouts. Bring to a boil and cook about 10 minutes. Dissolve cornstarch in small amount of cold water. Remove pot from heat. Gradually add cornstarch mixture, stirring well. Return to heat and stir until thickened. Serve immediately over brown rice.

Eat plenty of 100 percent whole wheat bread or rolls with this or any other meal if you like bread. Bread can make up your entire meal or snack.

    Servings: 6
    Preparation Time: 30 minutes
    Cooking Time: 5-10 minutes
      (Do not overcook)

Side Dish:
OVEN FRIED POTATOES
Wash and dry, but do not peel, 4 potatoes. Drop into a pot of boiling water, lower heat to simmer, and cook until barely tender. Remove from the pot and refrigerate. Alternate method-Microwave 4 potatoes for 15 minutes; don't overcook. Refrigerate. When potatoes are cool, peel them carefully and slice length-wise as for french fries. Spread the potatoes on a nonstick baking sheet and season with onion powder, garlic powder, paprika, black pepper, and/or chili powder. Brown in a 400° oven and turn with a spatula to brown the other side. Potatoes will be crispy.

    Servings: 4
    Preparation Time: 10 minutes   Cooking Time: 20-25 minutes

Dessert:

APPLE PIE

1 cup Grape-Nuts cereal, crushed
1/4 cup apple juice concentrate
1 can apples, packed in water
1/2 cup apple juice concentrate
1 tablespoon lemon juice
1 1/2 teaspoons apple pie spice, or
  1/2 teaspoon nutmeg, 1/4 teaspoon allspice, and 1 teaspoon cinnamon
1 tablespoon tapioca
2 tablespoons honey

For pie crust combine Grape-Nuts and 1/4 cup apple juice concentrate. Pat into a 9-inch pie pan. Place apples, concentrate, and tapioca in a saucepan; bring to a boil. Boil about 2 minutes. Stir in remaining ingredients. Pour into Grape-Nuts crust. Sprinkle a few crushed Grape-Nuts over top. Cover with foil and bake 1/2 hour at 350°.

Servings: 6
Preparation Time: 20 minutes
Cooking Time: 30 minutes

Day Six

Breakfast:

COLD CEREAL

1-3 cups of Shredded Wheat, Grape-Nuts, or any other acceptable cold
  cereal
1/4 cup sugar-free fruit juice
Fat-free Soy or Rice milk
1/2 banana, or 1/4 cup strawberries (optional)

Pour the cereal into a bowl, add the juice or milk; top with fruit if desired.

Servings: 1
Preparation Time: 2
Cooking Time: none

Lunch:
PINTO BEANS

Place 2 cups of cooked pinto beans in a bowl; microwave for 2-3 minutes, or heat in a saucepan on top of the stove over medium heat until hot. Serve with at least six raw vegetables and at least two slices of whole wheat bread. There are many brands of acceptable no-oil canned beans.

  Servings: 1
  Preparation Time: 2 minutes
  Cooking Time: none (if beans
    are pre-cooked)

Dinner:
SCALLOPED POTATOES

6 large potatoes cooked until almost tender, pared and thinly sliced
 (or about 5 cups)
2 medium thinly sliced onions
2 tablespoons flour
1 teaspoon salt (optional) salt to taste
1/8 teaspoon pepper
1 can defatted chicken broth or Swansons Chicken Broth,
   Fat-free, Cholesterol Free
Paprika

Arrange 1/3 of the potatoes in a 2 quart casserole. Arrange 1/3 of the onions on top of potatoes. Combine flour, salt and pepper. Sprinkle 1/3 of the flour mixture over potatoes and onions. Repeat layers twice. Pour chicken broth over all. Sprinkle with paprika. Cover, Bake at 375° for 15 minutes . Uncover and bake 30 minutes longer.

  Servings: 4-6
  Preparation Time: 20 minutes
  Cooking Time: 45 minutes

Salad:
CUCUMBER SALAD
1 medium cucumber, thinly sliced
1/2 cup thinly sliced red onion
1/2 cup New Kraft Fat-free Miracle Whip or Mayonnaise
Dash of salt
1/8 teaspoon pepper

Combine cucumber and onion slices in a bowl. Combine remaining ingredients and pour over slices. Toss and serve immediately.
   Servings: 4 (1/2 cup each)
   Preparation Time: 5 minutes
   Cooking Time: none

Vegetable:
CORN ON THE COB (OR FROZEN CORN KERNELS)
Shuck corn and place ears in a plastic bag. Place bag in the microwave oven: 1 ear, 4 minutes; 2 ears, 7 minutes; 3 ears, 11 minutes; and 4 ears, 14 minutes. Guard against burns when you remove the bag from the oven.
Alternate method: Place 4 inches of water in a large pot and bring to a boil. Drop the ear or ears of corn into boiling water and cook for 5-10 minutes. Don't overcook.
Frozen kernels cook quickly in a microwave oven—each cup of corn cooks in 2 or 3 minutes. Don't overcook. To cook frozen corn on top of the stove use very little water. Cover the bottom of the pan with 1/8 inch of water or less, and cook over medium heat for 3 to 5 minutes. Do not overcook.
   Servings: 1-4
   Preparation Time: 1-5 minutes
   Cooking Time: 4-14 minutes

Dessert:

FRUIT COBBLER

1 cup flour

1 cup sugar

1 cup non-fat soy milk

1 teaspoon baking powder

Mix together and pour into a 9"x13" non-stick baking dish. Sprinkle with Butter Buds and pour 1 quart fruit (With juice; blueberries, cherries, peaches, raspberries, etc.) on top of batter. Bake at 350° to 375° for 45 minutes.

NOTE: To use unsweetened pie cherries, use 1/4 to 1/2 cup sugar dissolved in the cherries before adding to batter.

   Servings: 10-12

   Preparation Time: 5-10 minutes

   Cooking Time: 40-45 minutes

Day Seven

Breakfast:

WHEATENA WHOLE WHEAT HOT CEREAL

Stovetop: Place 1 1/2 cups of water in saucepan. Add 1/2 cup Wheatena and heat to a rapid boil, stirring occasionally. Cook 4 to 5 minutes over moderate heat or to desired consistency, stirring occasionally. Remove from heat; cover until ready to serve. Stir before serving. Microwave instructions are on the box. Top off with an orange or banana.

   Servings: 1

   Preparation Time: 1 minute

   Cooking Time: 3-5 minutes

Lunch:

VEGETABLE STEW

(Recipe, pages 97 and 175)

Place 2 cups precooked vegetable stew in a saucepan or bowl. Heat on stovetop or in microwave oven for 2 to 3 minutes. Serve with two or more slices of whole-grain bread.

   Servings: 1

   Preparation Time: 1 minute

   Cooking Time: 2-3 minutes

Dinner:
BROCCOLI SURPRISE
1 16 oz bag frozen broccoli cuts
1 17 oz can creamed corn
1 cup non-fat milk thickened with 1 tablespoon cornstarch
Salt and pepper to taste
Butter Buds to taste
Thaw broccoli, but do not cook. Place in 2 quart casserole and sprinkle with salt and pepper lightly. Combine corn, milk, corn starch, and Butter Buds. Stir well. Pour over broccoli, sprinkle with bread crumbs. Bake at 350° 25-30 minutes or until firm and broccoli is tender.

    Servings: 4
    Preparation Time: 15 minutes
    Cooking Time: 30 minutes

Side Dish:
GREEN BEANS AND ONIONS
1 cup diced onions
4 cups cut canned green beans
1/2 teaspoon dill weed
Place the onions, beans, and dill weed in a saucepan. Add a small amount of water. Cook about 30 minutes.

    Servings: 6
    Preparation Time: 5-8 minutes
    Cooking Time: 30 minutes

Ditssert:

BAKED APPLES

4 apples, peeled
Apple pie spice
4 tablespoons undiluted frozen apple juice concentrate, thawed
4 teaspoons seedless raisins
Core apples; sprinkle apple pie spice into the core cavity. Fill each core with 1 tablespoon apple juice and 1 teaspoon raisins. Place apples in a small baking dish. Bake in a 350° oven for 1 hour or until the apples are fork tender.

Servings: 4

Preparation Time:15-20 minutes

Cooking Time: 1 hour

Repeat this seven-day menu for one more week, substituting with recipes in Chapter 20. After fourteen days on The Miracle Diet program, you will look and feel healthier. Adopting this eating program permanently will reduce your risk of suffering from heart disease, stroke, atherosclerosis, cancer, diabetes, and other diseases and allow you to enjoy the *"Best Possible Health."*

Twenty

Recipes for the "Best Possible Health"

Main Dishes

PIZZA

Sauce:

2 cups onions, diced	1 tablespoon garlic, minced
1 29-oz. can tomato sauce	1 teaspoon basil
1/2 teaspoon oregano	1/2 teaspoon salt
1/4 teaspoon pepper	1/8 teaspoon Tabasco sauce
1/8 teaspoon fennel seed	1/4 teaspoon thyme leaves

Place all ingredients in a medium saucepan. Simmer slowly for at least 60 minutes.

Crust:

1 cup bread flour	1 1/4 cup whole-wheat flour
1/4 cup gluten	1 pkg. rapid-rising yeast
1 teaspoon sugar	1 teaspoon salt (optional)
	1 1/4 cup hot water

Put crust ingredients in bread machine. Stop machine after first kneading. Let dough rest 15 minutes, then spread out in pizza pan. Add sauce and desired toppings such as bell peppers, green chiles, and mushrooms. Bake in non-stick pizza pan at 425° for 15 to 20 minutes.

Servings: 2 pizzas
Preparation Time: 30 minutes
Cooking Time: 15-20 minutes

100% WHOLE WHEAT-NO OIL PIZZA CRUST

2 1/4 cups whole wheat flour   1 teaspoon sugar
1/4 cup gluten   1 teaspoon salt (optional)'
1 pkg. rapid rising yeast   1 1/4 cup hot water

Put all ingredients in bread machine. Stop machine after first kneading. Let dough rest 15 minutes, then spread out in pizza pan. Add sauce and toppings. Use only plant food. Remember also olives are 99% fat.

If making without bread machine, knead full 15-20 minutes by hand. Let dough rest 15 minutes at least, then spread out in pizza pan. Add sauce and desired toppings. Bake 450⁰ for 15 to 20 minutes.

APPLE PIZZA

Recipe for pizza crust   1/3 cup brown sugar
4 medium apples (peeled & thinly sliced)   1 teaspoon cinnamon

Prepare pizza crust as per recipe. Pat dough into a pizza pan or a baking sheet. Crimp edges as for a pizza. Spread apples over dough and sprinkle brown sugar and cinnamon over apples. Bake at 425⁰ for 30 minutes.

POTATO CASSEROLE DINNER

6 potatoes, sliced   2 onions, sliced
1 green pepper, sliced   2 carrots, sliced
1 cup fresh or frozen green peas   1 cup fresh or frozen corn
1 zucchini, sliced   1/2 cup broccoli
1 cup green beans (optional)

Sauce:
3 cups tomato sauce   1 teaspoon ground thyme
2 tablespoons low-salt soy sauce   1/8 teaspoon oregano
2 teaspoons parsley flakes   1 teaspoon chili powder
1 teaspoon dry mustard

Layer the vegetables in a large casserole dish in the order given. Mix sauce ingredients; pour over layered vegetables. Bake, covered, in a 350° oven for approximately 1 1/2 hours. This dish can be prepared ahead for a company dinner. Serve with whole-grain bread and a mixed green salad.

Servings: 8
Preparation Time: 30 minutes
Cooking Time: 1 1/2 hours

MARILYN'S VEGETABLE STIR FRY

1 Green pepper, cut into 1" squares	Snow peas, washed and trimmed
1/2 cup fresh mushrooms, sliced	1/2 cup celery, sliced diagonally
1 small can water chestnuts, drained	About 1 cup broccoli florets
About 1/2 cup cauliflower florets	2-3 cloves garlic, minced

1 onion, layers separated and cut into 1 " squares
1 carrot cut into slices 1" square 1/8" thick (par-boil carrots in saucepan)
About 1" fresh ginger root, peeled and minced
2 tablespoons cornstarch mixed in 1/2 cup cold water
1/2 cup low sodium soy sauce
Several green onions cut into 1" pieces and sliced lengthwise (save for topping)

Put several tablespoons water in heated wok or skillet. Cook the onion first until transparent. Then add broccoli and anything else that might benefit from a couple extra minutes of cooking. Put the lid on the wok and steam for a couple of minutes, then add remaining vegetables, stirring constantly. Do not overcook. At the last, add soy sauce to cornstarch mixture and add to vegetables; keep stirring and add additional soy sauce if needed for desired consistency of sauce.
Sprinkle green onions on top, serve immediately over hot brown rice.

    Servings: 6
    Preparation Time: 30 minutes
    Cooking Time: 10 minutes

BROWN GRAVY ON MASHED POTATOES

1/4 cup water	1 cup whole wheat flour
1 onion, finely chopped	5 cups water
1/4 cup low-salt soy sauce	

1/2 pound sliced mushrooms, or 8-oz. can mushrooms

Heat 1/4 cup water in large saucepan over medium heat; add onion and saute for 5 minutes, until translucent. Blend in flour and stir well. Cook for 3 to 4 minutes, until lightly browned. Add the water and soy sauce. Stir until blended well. Add mushrooms and cook over medium heat, stirring often, until sauce thickens. Add more water if too thick. Serve over mashed potatoes.

    Servings: 6-8
    Preparation Time: 10 minutes
    Cooking Time: 10 minutes

CHILI

2 1/2 cups dried pinto beans
1 cup brown rice
7 1/2 cups water
2 green peppers, chopped
3 onions, chopped
1 tablespoon low-salt soy sauce
1 28-oz. can tomatoes, cut up, or 2 cups chopped fresh tomatoes
6 cloves garlic, crushed
3 teaspoons chili powder
1 teaspoon cumin (optional)
1 cup corn kernels

Place beans, rice, and water in a large pot. Cover and cook over fairly low heat, about 1 1/2 hours. The vegetables, spices, and tomatoes can be prepared while the beans and rice are beginning to cook. After 90 minutes, add remaining ingredients except corn kernels to the pot. Cook 2 more hours; uncover during the last 30 minutes of cooking and add the corn kernels. Can be cooked longer than 3 1/2 hours if desired. Makes excellent leftovers; spoon into pita bread or over corn chips. Note: Soaking beans overnight cuts down on cooking time.

    Servings: 8
    Preparation Time: 30 minutes
    Cooking Time: 3 1/2 hours

DILLED POTATOES

4 medium potatoes, peeled and quartered
2 small onions, diced
2 cups water
1/4 teaspoon Mrs. Dash
1/4 teaspoon dill weed
Dash of black pepper
Dash of cayenne pepper

Place potatoes in a saucepan with water, dill weed, onion, and peppers. Simmer, covered, over low heat for 15 minutes or until potatoes are tender.

    Servings: 4
    Preparation Time: 10 minutes
    Cooking Time: 15 minutes

ETHEL'S PINTO BEANS

4 cups pinto beans (soak overnight then pour water off and rinse)
2 chopped onions
1/4 to 1/2 teaspoons garlic powder
1 to 3 teaspoons salt (optional)
1/2 cup ketchup
1/4 teaspoon black pepper

Bring beans to boil, then pour off water. Rinse and place in pressure cooker along with all other ingredients. Add water approximately 2" above beans. Bring up pressure on pressure cooker, and turn heat to medium-low. Cook for 1 1/2 hours. Turn off heat and allow pressure to escape on its own. (Never fill pressure cooker over 3/4 full with food or liquid.) Without using pressure, allow about 4 hours cooking time.

    Servings: 12
    Preparation Time: 15 minutes
    Cooking Time: 1 1/2 hours

LIMA BEANS AND PASTA

3 cups uncooked whole wheat pasta
3 stalks celery, sliced
3 cups uncooked lima beans (soak overnight, then pour water off and rinse)
3 onions, chopped
8 cups water
2 cloves garlic, crushed or 1/2 teaspoon garlic powder
3/4 teaspoon thyme
3/4 teaspoon basil
1 1/2 tablespoons low salt soy sauce

Bring beans to a boil in a large pot, then pour off water. Bring beans to a boil again, lower heat, cover pot and simmer at low heat 1/2 hour. Add other ingredients, except pasta. Cook 45 minutes longer. Add the pasta and cook until tender, about 10-15 minutes.

    Servings: 8
    Preparation Time: 15 minutes
    Cooking Time: 1 1/2 hours

BEANS WITH BARLEY

6 cups cooked pinto beans
3 cups cooked barley
1 onion, chopped
1 small can mushrooms
1/4 teaspoon rosemary

2 cups chopped spinach
1 tablespoon low-salt soy sauce
1 tablespoon lemon juice
1 cup water

Place all ingredients in a large pot. Bring to a boil, turn heat to medium and cook for 30 minutes.

Servings: 6-8
Preparation Time: 15 minutes
Cooking Time: 30 minutes

MEXICAN CHILI BEANS

Cook your own dry pinto beans, because you need the cooking liquid from the beans to make good chili. Soaking the beans overnight cuts cooking time in half.

4 cups dry pinto beans
10 cups water
2 green peppers, chopped
4 yellow onions, chopped
4 cloves garlic, crushed
2 cups tomato sauce
2 16-oz. cans tomatoes, cut up, or stewed tomatoes

8 tablespoons chili powder
3 teaspoons ground cumin
1/2 teaspoon crushed red pepper
1/4 teaspoon cayenne pepper
4 stalks celery, chopped

Place the pinto beans and water in a 6-quart pot. Bring to a boil. Pour off water and replace; bring to a boil again, reduce heat, and simmer for 2 hours. Add the remaining ingredients and cook an additional 2 hours or more until beans are soft. Serve over brown rice if desired. Freeze all left-over chili for a quick meal later.

Servings: 8-10
Preparation Time: 15 minutes
Cooking Time: 4 hours

REFRIED BEANS

6 cups cooked pinto beans   1/2 teaspoon chili powder
1/4 teaspoon garlic powder   1/2 cup picante sauce or salsa
1/2 teaspoon onion powder   1/2 cup bean-water or water

Mash cooked beans with water until desired consistency is reached. Add
onion powder, garlic powder, and chili powder. Mix well. Stir in salsa; cook
over low heat about 15 minutes, or until heated through. Serve in bean enchiladas, on tostados, in pita bread, or with home-baked corn chips.
   Servings: 8-10
   Preparation Time: 5 minutes
   Cooking Time: 20 minutes

BEANS AND RICE

1 cup cooked beans (any variety, no-oil)   1 cup cooked brown rice

Mix cooked beans and rice together in a bowl, heat in microwave oven for 2-
3 minutes. Makes an excellent quick meal anytime and cuts down on the
high protein of beans alone. For variety, try ketchup, hot sauce, red pepper
or other seasonings.
Eat a salad of five or six cut raw vegetables and whole wheat bread or cornbread for a complete meal.
   Servings: Variable
   Preparation Time: 2-3 minutes
   Cooking Time: 2-3 minutes

BEAN BURRITOS

Cooked pinto beans   Whole wheat flour tortillas
Hot sauce (per next recipe)   Cilantro leaves seasoning
Diced lettuce, tomatoes and green onions

Drain juice from pinto beans and mash by hand or use blender. Place a tortilla on plate. Spoon a layer of beans and hot sauce into center of tortilla.
Sprinkle cilantro (use sparingly) and green onions over beans and sauce.
Roll up tortilla, place in foil and heat through. After heating remove foil and
place on a warm plate. Add a little hot sauce over top and top with lettuce
and tomatoes.

HOT SAUCE

1 29-oz can tomato puree	1 1/2 teaspoon chili powder
3/8 teaspoon oregano	3/4 teaspoon garlic powder
3/8 teaspoon Tabasco sauce	3/8 teaspoon cumin
4 1/2 teaspoon lemon juice	3/8 teaspoon salt
3/8 teaspoon black pepper	3/8 teaspoon red pepper
1 teaspoon red wine vinegar	

Combine all ingredients. Keeps well in refrigerator for up to 2 weeks and freezes well. Makes a wonderful chip dip.

   Preparation Time: 15 minutes
   Cooking Time: None

BAKED BROWN RICE

1 cup brown rice
3 teaspoons minced onion
1 teaspoon dehydrated parsley
2 1/2 cups defatted beef broth*
1 teaspoon Mrs. Dash

Brown the rice in a nonstick skillet. When golden brown, place in tightly covered casserole. Pour over rice, 2 1/2 cups of hot defatted beef broth* (mix as per directions on can). Bake in a 350° oven for one hour. Garnish with dehydrated parsley. Add more water if needed during cooking. *(To remove fat, chill can of beef broth in refrigerator; lift off congealed fat with spoon)

   Servings: 4-6
   Preparation Time: 10 minutes
   Cooking Time: 1 hour

SPANISH RICE

2 cups uncooked brown rice
3 1/2 cups water
1/2 cup chopped celery
1 teaspoon parsley flakes
1/4 teaspoon Mrs. Dash
1 29-oz. can tomato sauce

1/2 cup chopped onions
1/2 cup chopped green pepper
1/8 teaspoon ground pepper
1/4 teaspoon garlic powder
1/8 teaspoon oregano
1/4 teaspoon cumin

In a nonstick pan, stir the brown rice over medium heat to toast the rice evenly. Add all ingredients and mix well. Simmer covered for about 1 hour or until all liquid is absorbed. Place in 3 quart covered casserole dish and bake at 350° F. until desired tenderness. Small amount of water may be added if necessary.

Servings: 6-8
Preparation Time: 30 minutes
Cooking Time: 1 1/2 hour

GLORIFIED ZUCCHINI

2 zucchini, thinly sliced
2 stalks celery, sliced
1 cup water
1/8 teaspoon ground pepper
1/2 pound fresh mushrooms, sliced
1 onion, sliced
1/2 teaspoon dried thyme
1 teaspoon Mrs. Dash

Place zucchini, mushrooms, celery, onion, Mrs. Dash, and water in saucepan. Add the thyme and pepper. Simmer, covered, 15 to 20 minutes or until tender.

Servings: 4-6
Preparation Time: 15 minutes
Cooking Time: 15-20 minutes

MACARONI GARDEN SALAD

4 cups cooked egg-free macaroni
1/4 teaspoon dry mustard
1/4 teaspoon pepper
6 green onions, chopped fine
1 large bell pepper, chopped
1/2 cup Kraft Fat-Free Mayonnaise or Miracle Whip
2 teaspoons dill weed

3 teaspoons Mrs. Dash	1/4 cup chopped parsley
2 stalks celery, chopped	1 cucumber, chopped
1 large tomato, chopped	4-5 tablespoons dice pimiento
1 cup cooked green peas	1/2 cup oil-free Italian dressing

Mix Miracle Whip, mustard, and dill weed. Pour over cooled, cooked macaroni. Mix well, add remaining ingredients. Toss gently. Cover and refrigerate at least 2 hours before serving.

   Servings: 6
   Preparation Time: 30 minutes
   Cooking Time: none

CORN BREAD SALAD

1 pan baked no-fat cornbread
2 small jars chopped pimientos
2 large tomatoes, diced
1 1/2 cups Kraft Fat-Free Miracle Whip or Fat-Free Mayonnaise
1 1/2 cups sweet onions, chopped fine
3 stalks celery, chopped
2 large chopped bell peppers
1 cup chopped green onions with stems

Crumble cornbread; mix in vegetables and Mayonnaise. Chill. Keeps several days in refrigerator. (A little purple onion and/or black pepper can be added for color and extra flavor.)

   Servings: 6
   Preparation Time: 20 minutes
   Cooking Time: none

RICE DELIGHT

1 cup uncooked brown rice
2 1/2 cups water
1 medium, chopped onion

1 2-oz. jar pimientos
1 4-oz. can chopped green chiles
1/2 teaspoon Mrs. Dash

Place 2 1/2 cups of water in 3-quart saucepan; bring to a boil. Add rice, cover pan, and turn heat to low. Cook until all the water is absorbed (approx. 1 hour). Add remaining ingredients and cook another 5 minutes.

Servings: 4-6
Preparation Time: 10 minutes
Cooking Time: 1 hour

RICE SUBLIME

1 cup uncooked brown rice
1 1/2 cups frozen green peas
2 cups sliced fresh mushrooms
1 small jar pimientos
1/4 teaspoon garlic powder
1/8 teaspoon black pepper

2 1/2 cups water
1 onion, chopped
1 8-oz. can water chestnuts
1/4 cup low-sodium soy sauce
1/2 teaspoon Mrs. Dash

Mix rice, water, onion, mushrooms, and seasonings together. Bring to a boil, lower heat, and cook 45 minutes. Add green peas, pimiento, and water chestnuts. Cook an additional 15 minutes.

Servings: 4
Preparation Time: 15 minutes
Cooking Time: 1 hour

CHILI RICE VERDE

4 cups cooked brown rice
1 4 oz. can chopped green chilies
1 cup non-fat soy milk
1 tablespoon cornstarch
Dash pepper and salt
1/2 cup shredded no-fat Smart Beat (New, looks like cheese slices, non-dairy) (optional)

Mix milk and cornstarch. Combine all ingredients, place in 2 quart covered casserole dish and bake 30 minutes at 350° F.
Servings: 4
Preparation Time: 10 minutes
Cooking Time: 30 minutes

MUSHROOM CURRY RICE

1/2 lb. fresh mushrooms, sliced
1 medium onion, chopped
2 medium apples, chopped
1 teaspoon curry powder
1/2 teaspoon Mrs. Dash
3 cups Fat-free Miracle Whip
2 cups cooked brown rice
Paprika
Salt to taste (optional)

Slice mushrooms, chop onion and apples. Saute vegetables in 1/2 cup of water till tender crisp. In small bowl mix Miracle Whip, curry powder, Mrs. Dash, salt. Place vegetables over the top of rice. Place the mixture on top of vegetables and sprinkle with paprika. Bake at 350° for 30 minutes. Add raisins for variety.
Servings: 4-6
Preparation Time: 20 minutes
Cooking Time: 30 minutes

STIR FRY WITH TVP

TVP Preparation

1 cup water
2 teaspoons beef bouillon
1 cup TVP beef-style strips

In a small saucepan bring 1 cup water to a boil. Add TVP and beef bouillon. Remove from heat and let stand 10 minutes.

Remaining Ingredients

1 tablespoon cornstarch
3 tablespoons rice vinegar
1/4 cup lite soy sauce
1/4 cup water
1/2 tablespoon sugar
1/4 teaspoon red pepper
1/2 teaspoon ground ginger
1 clove garlic, minced
1 pound fresh broccoli, sliced
1 cup fresh cauliflower, sliced
1 white onion, sliced
2 stalks celery, sliced
1/2 red bell pepper, julienned
1/2 green bell pepper, julienned

TVP: Soybean product, 4% fat. Replaces meat, high in protein, 52%. Available from:
Harvest Direct
P.O. Box 4514
Decatur, IL 62525
1 (800) 835-2867

Optional Ingredients

1 can (5 oz.) water chestnuts, drained
1 can mushrooms (4 oz.)
2 cups bean sprouts (fresh)

Prepare vegetables before starting to cook. Combine rice vinegar, soy sauce, 1/4 cup water, sugar, red pepper and cornstarch, mix well and set aside.

In a wok or large skillet pour 1/4 cup water. Stir in ginger and garlic and saute for one minute. Add TVP, broccoli and cauliflower and continue cooking for 3 minutes. Add onion, celery and bell pepper. Cook 3 more minutes. Add cornstarch mixture, continue cooking for 3 minutes. Add any or all optional ingredients and cook one more minute. Serve immediately. Serve with rice for a complete meal.

> Preparation time: 30 minutes
> Cooking time: 10 minutes
> Servings: 4-6

BEAN TOSTADOS-BEAN BURRITOS

Layer tostada as follows: Lay a whole wheat flour or non-fat corn tortilla flat on serving plate. Spoon on 4 or 5 tablespoons of precooked pinto beans (see recipe below) down the center of the tortilla. Add shredded lettuce, chopped tomatoes, alfalfa sprouts, salsa or hot sauce, and a pinch of dry cilantro leaves. To make burrito, fold the tortilla over the ingredients. Can be eaten with a fork or picked up and eaten as a sandwich. There are many variations, experiment.

    Servings: Variable
    Preparation Time: 15 minutes
    Cooking Time: none

Pinto Beans:

Soak 2 cups dry pinto beans (can also use black beans) overnight in about 4 cups of water. After soaking, keep just enough water to cover beans and add 1 14-oz. can of clear beef broth from which fat had been removed. (To remove fat, chill can of beef broth in the refrigerator; lift off congealed fat.) Cook beans until tender (about 3 hours) with:

1/2 teaspoon garlic (or crushed clove garlic)
1/2 cup finely chopped onion
1 teaspoon cumin
Dash of salt (optional)

Mash beans before serving. Beans store well in the refrigerator (about one week) or freezer.

    Servings: 8-10
    Preparation Time: 10 minutes
    Cooking Time: none

Soups

CREAM OF BROCCOLI SOUP

1 10-oz. package chopped broccoli
1/2 teaspoon minced garlic
1 small onion, diced
1 teaspoon Mrs. Dash
1/2 teaspoon curry powder
1 cup non-fat soy milk
1 cup water
3 tablespoons flour
1 tablespoon lemon juice

Place broccoli, onion, and garlic in saucepan with water. Cover and cook until very soft. Combine 1 cup of soy milk and flour in a jar and shake until smooth. Add milk and flour mixture to broccoli mixture. Add remaining ingredients and cook until thick, stirring constantly. Serve immediately.

Servings: 2
Preparation Time: 25 minutes
Cooking Time: 25 minutes

ONION BARLEY SOUP

6 cups defatted beef broth (to remove fat, chill can of broth in refrigerator; lift off congealed fat with spoon)
4 onions, sliced
1 cup cooked barley
2 tablespoons (low-sodium) soy sauce
1/2 teaspoon dry mustard
1/2 teaspoon thyme leaves
1/2 teaspoon garlic powder

Saute onions in 1/2 cup water. Cook about 15 minutes or until soft and tender. Add beef broth and barley. Bring to a boil. Add seasonings. Reduce heat to low and simmer covered about 30 minutes before serving.

Servings: 6
Preparation Time: 15 minutes
Cooking Time: 30 minutes

LIMA BEAN SOUP

1 1/2 cups dried lima beans
1 bay leaf
1 1/2 cups chopped carrots
1/2 cup finely chopped green pepper
1 1/2 cups chopped celery
1 1/2 cups chopped onions
1 1/2 cans cut green beans
1 cup canned tomatoes, chopped small
1/2 teaspoon black pepper
2 teaspoons basil
1 teaspoon Mrs. Dash
Water as required

Rinse and soak beans overnight. Drain. Cover with water to about 3 inches above surface of the beans. Add bay leaf and cook until tender. Replenish the water in the bean pot to about 3 inches above the surface. Add the celery, carrots, onions, green peppers, and green beans. Add more water as required. Toward the end of the cooking period, when the vegetables are almost tender, add seasonings and chopped tomatoes. Discard bay leaf.

Servings: 6-8
Preparation Time: 30 minutes
Cooking Time: 2 1/4 hours

SPLIT PEA SOUP

2 cups dry split peas
2 quarts water
1 onion, finely diced
2 carrots, finely diced
1 teaspoon parsley flakes

2 celery stalks, diced
1/4 teaspoon pepper
1 bay leaf
1/4 teaspoon Mrs. Dash

Soak peas in water overnight; drain. Rinse once and add 2 quarts of water. Bring to a boil; reduce heat, cover, and cook until tender (2 hours or more). Add the remaining ingredients and simmer for 1 hour. Discard bay leaf. Add extra pepper or red pepper if desired.

Servings: 8-10
Preparation Time: 15 minutes
Cooking Time: 2-3 hours

BARLEY MUSHROOM SOUP

4 cups cooked barley
4 cups water
1 cup diced celery
2 large diced onions
1/2 teaspoon garlic powder
1 teaspoon basil leaves
1/4 teaspoon paprika
1/4 teaspoon chili powder
1 teaspoon Mrs. Dash
    1 teaspoon oregano

4 cups defatted beef broth*
6 cups sliced mushrooms
1 cup finely diced carrots
4 teaspoons worcestershire
  sauce
1/2 teaspoon thyme
1 teaspoon parsley flakes
1 teaspoon dill weed
1 teaspoon salt (optional)

Saute vegetables in 1 cup water. Combine all ingredients and simmer at least one hour.

*(To remove fat, chill can of beef broth in refrigerator; lift off congealed fat with spoon)

    Preparation Time: 30 minutes
    Cooking Time: 1 hour

CREAM OF CORN SOUP

4 cups cooked frozen corn
4 cups fat-free soy milk mixed well with 4 tablespoons
  cornstarch or flour
1/2 teaspoon dill weed
1 teaspoon Mrs. Dash
1/4 teaspoon black pepper

Put corn in a blender and process until slightly chopped. Empty the corn into a saucepan; add the milk, dill weed, and pepper. Stir well and heat for several minutes, until slightly thick.

    Servings: 4-6
    Preparation Time: 10 minutes
    Cooking Time: 10-15 minutes

VEGETABLE NOODLE SOUP

1 14-oz can defatted chicken broth or
  Swanson Chicken Broth (fat-free, low salt)

4 sliced carrots	1 cup mini noodle
1 large diced onion	3 stalks diced celery
1 teaspoon basil leaves	1 small can sliced mushrooms
1/2 teaspoon thyme leaves	1/2 teaspoon garlic powder
1 teaspoon parsley flakes	1/8 teaspoon black pepper
1/8 teaspoon paprika	1 teaspoon salt (optional)
1/4 teaspoon dill weed	1/4 teaspoon chili powder

Saute carrots, celery, and onion in 1/2 cup water. Add chicken broth and all other ingredients. Simmer for at least one hour.

    Servings: 6
    Preparation Time: 30 minutes
    Cooking Time: 1 hour

10-BEAN SOUP

4 cups 10-bean soup mix
1 large onion, chopped
4 quarts water
1 clove garlic, minced
1 16-oz. can tomatoes, undrained and chopped
1 sm. can green chilies (optional)
1 1/2 teaspoons Mrs. Dash

Sort and wash bean mix. In a large pot, soak beans overnight in 2 inches of water. Drain beans; add 4 quarts of water and add onion, garlic and Mrs. Dash. Cover and bring to a boil; reduce heat and simmer 2 hours or until beans are tender. Add tomatoes and chilies; simmer 30 minutes longer, stirring occasionally.

    Servings: 10-12
    Preparation Time: 10 minutes
    Cooking Time: 3-4 hours

LAURA'S CREAM OF POTATO SOUP

5 or 6 medium potatoes, peeled and cubed
6 cups water
1 medium onion, diced, or 1 tablespoon onion powder
1 stalk celery, diced, or 1 tablespoon celery flakes or
  1/8 teaspoon celery seed
1/8 teaspoon garlic powder
1 bay leaf
1 teaspoon salt (optional)
1/8 teaspoon pepper
1/8 teaspoon dill weed
1/16 teaspoon or dash paprika
1 teaspoon parsley flakes
2 tablespoons flour mixed in 1/2 cup water until smooth

Place all ingredients in large saucepan. Cook until potatoes are very tender. Remove 1/3 to 1/2 of the potatoes to a bowl and mash well. Remove and discard bay leaf. Return mashed potatoes to pan. Thicken soup to desired consistency with flour mixture.

Servings: 6
Preparation Time: 25 minutes
Cooking Time: 55 minutes

BLACK BEAN SOUP

2 cups black beans
2 tablespoons red wine vinegar
6-8 cups water
1/2 teaspoon dried thyme
2 onions, chopped
1/2 teaspoon dried oregano
1 clove garlic, minced

2 tablespoons low-sodium soy sauce
2 cups chopped tomatoes
1 cup chopped celery
1/2 cup chopped green onion
1 tablespoon jalapeno pepper
2 tablespoons salsa

Soak beans overnight; rinse. Cook beans in water with the chopped onion and garlic for 2 hours or until tender. Add tomato, celery, green pepper, jalapeno pepper, red wine vinegar, thyme, oregano, and soy sauce. Continue cooking for 1 hour or more. Serve with 1 tablespoon chopped green onions and a helping of salsa.

Servings: 10 cups
Preparation Time: 15 minutes   Cooking Time: 3 or 4 hours

4-GRAIN SOUP

10 cups water	1/2 cup whole wheat berries
2/3 cup lentils	1/2 cup brown rice
1/4 cup barley	1/4 cup parsley flakes
1 tablespoon onion powder	1/2 tablespoon garlic powder
1 teaspoon basil	1/2 teaspoon cumin
1 1/2 cups chopped onion	1/2 cup sliced carrots
1/2 cup sliced celery	1/2 cup cubed potatoes
3 tablespoons low-sodium soy sauce	1 cup frozen corn kernels
1 cup frozen peas	

Place the water in a large soup pot. Add wheat berries, lentils, brown rice, barley, parsley, and spices. Bring to a boil and cook over medium heat for 60 minutes. Add the fresh chopped vegetables; cook additional 20 minutes. Add the frozen vegetables and cook an additional 10 minutes.

Servings: 8-10
Preparation Time: 30 minutes
Cooking Time: 1 1/2 hours

VEGETABLE SOUP (STEW)

4 potatoes, cut in medium-sized chunks	1/2 cup frozen corn
1 46 oz. can tomato juice	1/2 teaspoon Mrs. Dash-herbs
4 medium onion, sliced small	1 cup pearled barley
1 28 oz. can tomatoes	1/2 teaspoon dill weed
4 large stalks of celery, sliced	4 large carrots, sliced
1/4 teaspoon pepper, dash of red pepper	
1/2 cup sliced frozen okra, frozen broccoli, or both	

In a six-quart pan add the can of tomato juice to the cut vegetables. Add the can of tomatoes, and cut up the tomatoes. Add 1 cup of water. Bring to a boil. Add seasonings. Simmer over medium-low heat about 30 to 45 minutes. Do not over-cook. The carrots should be crunchy. Cook the barley separately and add about 15 minutes before end of cooking time. Add 1/2 cup of corn in the last 3 minutes of cooking time. You may want to use 1 cup of cooked brown rice or broken up whole-wheat spaghetti as options in place of the barley. This recipe will make enough for several meals.

Helpful hints: Other vegetables may be used in addition to or in place of the ones listed above. Try 1/2 cup of frozen peas, chopped spinach, sliced mushrooms, or one green pepper added during the last 4 minutes of cooking time.

Sandwiches

TOMATO BURGER

1 burger bun
1 to 4 tomato slices
1 onion slice
1 lettuce leaf
4 pickle slices
fat-free mayonnaise and/or mustard

Spread mayonnaise and/or mustard on bun; arrange other ingredients and enjoy!
> Yield: 1 burger
> Preparation Time: 5 minutes

Note: Order this at your favorite fast food chain.

BEAN BURGER

1 burger bun
1/2 cup canned fat-free refried beans
1 slice red onion
1 slice tomato
1 lettuce leaf
fat-free mayonnaise or mustard to taste
1 Tbsp. salsa (optional)

Put all ingredients on a bun and *presto* you have a bean burger
> Yield: 1 burger
> Preparation Time: 5 minutes

BOCA BURGER
(fat-free)

A delicious alternative to the high-cholesterol, high-fat animal-food hamburger

1 Boca Burger pattie
1 slice tomato
1 lettuce leaf
1 slice onion
1 burger bun
garnish with pickles

Brown pattie in a non-stick skillet. Assemble like a hamburger.
    Servings: 1 burger per person
    Preparation Time: 5 minutes
    Cooking Time: 5 minutes

Note: Fat-free Boca Burgers can be purchased in most health food stores. If they don't carry this item, ask them to order the product for you. This is a frozen product from Boca Raton, Florida.

GRILLED CHEESE SANDWICH

1 slice Smart Beat® Lactose Free Cheese
2 slices whole wheat bread
1 slice tomato
1 lettuce leaf

Put cheese between slices of bread and brown in non-stick skillet. (You may want to lightly spray skillet with no-stick cooking spray) when cheese is soft open sandwich and add tomato and lettuce. WOW! You have a lactose free, fat and cholesterol free, non-dairy cheese sandwich. Serve with pickles and baked chips for a hearty lunch.
    Yield: 1 sandwich
    Preparation Time: 5 minutes
    Cooking Time: 5 minutes

Sauces

MEXICAN HOT SAUCE OR DIP

1 29-oz can tomato puree
3/8 teaspoon oregano
2 teaspoons lemon juice
3/8 teaspoon black pepper
1 1/2 teaspoons chili powder
3/4 teaspoon garlic powder
3/8 teaspoon Tabasco sauce
3/8 teaspoon cumin
3/8 teaspoon salt
3/8 teaspoon red pepper
1 1/2 teaspoons red wine vinegar

Combine all ingredients. Keeps well in refrigerator for up to 2 weeks and freezes well. Makes a wonderful chip dip.
    Servings: variable
    Preparation Time: 15 minutes
    Cooking Time: None

SWEET AND SOUR SAUCE

1/2 cup unsweetened pineapple juice
2 cups peeled and chopped apples
2 tablespoons cider vinegar
2 tablespoons honey
1 teaspoon low-sodium soy sauce

Combine all ingredients in a saucepan. Cover and cook until fruit is tender, about 20 minutes. Mash with a hand masher. If you want a thicker sauce add 1 tablespoon of cornstarch to the liquid before cooking and stir well until thick. Serve hot or cold.
    Servings: makes 2 cups
    Preparation Time: 15 minutes
    Cooking Time: 20 minutes

BROWN GRAVY

2 cups cold water
7 tablespoons whole wheat flour
1 teaspoon minced onion
1/4 teaspoon onion powder
1/8 teaspoon garlic powder
1 tablespoon low-sodium soy sauce

Combine water and flour. Stir until well blended. Cook over low heat until thickened, approximately 10 minutes. Add remaining ingredients. Continue to cook over low heat for 10 minutes, stirring occasionally.

Servings: makes 2 cups
Preparation Time: 5 minutes
Cooking Time: 20 minutes

CREAMED MUSHROOM SAUCE

1/2 pound sliced mushrooms
1 onion, chopped
2 cups fat-free soy milk
1/8 teaspoon white pepper
1/8 teaspoon garlic powder
1 tablespoon low-sodium soy sauce
2 tablespoons cornstarch

Saute the onions and the mushrooms in 1/4 cup water for 10 minutes. Add milk, garlic powder, soy sauce, and white pepper. Mix cornstarch in 1/4 cup cold water. Add to mushroom mixture. Cook and stir over medium heat until mixture thickens. Great over grains, potatoes, vegetables, and rice.

Servings: makes 3 cups
Preparation Time: 15 minutes
Cooking Time: 25 minutes

FANTASTIC SPAGHETTI SAUCE

2 cans (28-oz.) tomatoes, slightly chopped
2 cans (29-oz.) tomato sauce
3 cups chopped onion
2 cups chopped bell pepper
5 or 6 cups sliced mushrooms
1 tablespoon garlic, minced
2 tablespoons wine vinegar
2 tablespoons basil
2 teaspoons Mrs. Dash mixed spices and herbs

Combine all ingredients, except basil, in a large saucepan or skillet. Simmer about 1 hour; add basil and simmer 30 minutes longer. You can make the sauce early in the day and reheat just before serving. About 15 minutes before serving, drop 1 pound of egg-free whole wheat or spinach spaghetti into 4 quarts boiling water and cook until tender, or about 10 minutes. Serve with sauce. Freeze leftover sauce for future use.

Servings: 10-12
Preparation Time: 15 minutes
Cooking Time: 1 1/2 hours

ENCHILADA SAUCE

2 onion, chopped
1 4 oz. can chopped green chilies
1/2 teaspoon basil
1/4 teaspoon ground oregano
1 tablespoon soy sauce

2 cloves garlic, crushed
3 1/2 cups tomato sauce
1/8 teaspoon ground cumin
1 1/2 cups water
4 tablespoons cornstarch

In a large saucepan saute onions and garlic in 1/4 cup of the water for 10 minutes. Blend the tomato sauce with green chili and seasonings. Simmer for about 20 minutes. Stir soy sauce into 1 cup water and add to the tomato sauce mixture. Dissolve cornstarch in remaining 1/4 cup water and add to the tomato sauce mixture. Simmer about 15 minutes longer over low heat stirring often. Serve over bean enchiladas or rice dishes.

Servings: 6
Preparation Time: 15 minutes
Cooking Time: 30-45 minutes

Salads

SPINACH SALAD

1 large bunch spinach
6 florets cauliflower
4 ozs. mushrooms, washed and sliced
1 onion, thinly sliced
No-oil Italian or Herb dressing

Wash and stem spinach. Dry. Tear into pieces. Thinly slice cauliflower florets. Combine first four ingredients and serve with dressing.

Servings: 4
Preparation Time: 30 minutes
Cooking Time: none

FRUIT SALAD

Apple chunks		Peach slices		Watermelon chunks
Banana chunks	or	Pear slices	or	Honeydew chunks
Pineapple chunks		Orange sections		Cantaloupe chunks
Strawberries		Banana slices		Grapes

Serve ice-cold and garnish each dish with a sprig of mint.

Preparation Time: 15 minutes

CUCUMBER-TOMATO-ONION SALAD

4 ounces Kraft Fat-free Mayonnaise
1 large cucumber, peeled and sliced thin
4 tomatoes, sliced   1/4 teaspoon dill
2 onions, sliced thin   Pepper to taste
1/4 cup apple cider vinegar

Layer the slices of vegetables in a bowl. Pour the vinegar and mayo over them. Chill until served.

Servings: 4
Preparation Time: 15 minutes

SLICED TOMATO SALAD

2 large tomatoes
Fresh parsley
1 small mild onion
Fat-free Italian dressing

Slice tomatoes and onions onto individual salad plates. Sprinkle lightly with pepper and Italian dressing. Garnish with parsley.
   Servings: 4
   Preparation Time: 10 minutes

COLESLAW

4 cups shredded cabbage
1 medium carrot, shredded
1 onion, finely chopped
Dash of salt
1/2 cup Kraft Fat-Free Miracle Whip or Mayonnaise
Dash of paprika

Combine all ingredients except paprika; sprinkle paprika on top.
   Servings: 6
   Preparation Time: 20 minutes
   Cooking Time: none

CARROT-RAISIN SALAD

4 carrots, grated/shredded
1/4 cup raisins
4 oz. crushed pineapple with juice (1/2 small can)

Mix all ingredients well. To blend flavors better, refrigerate a few hours before serving.
   Servings: 4
   Preparation Time: 5-10 minutes
   Cooking Time: none

CUCUMBER SALAD

1 medium cucumber, thinly sliced
1/2 cup thinly sliced red onion
1/2 cup plain, Kraft Fat-free Mayonnaise
Dash of salt
1/8 teaspoon pepper

Combine cucumber and onion slices in a bowl. Combine remaining ingredients and pour over slices. Toss and serve immediately.
    Servings: 4 (1/2 cup each)
    Preparation Time: 5 minutes
    Cooking Time: none

POTATO SALAD

6 cups diced cooked potatoes
1 or 2 medium chopped onions
1 tablespoon mustard
1/2 cup diced celery
    Salt and pepper to taste
1 cup Kraft Fat-free
  Mayonnaise
  or Miracle Whip
3/4 cup sweet pickle relish

Combine all ingredients; mix well. Better if chilled for an hour before serving. For extra color, sprinkle with a little paprika.
    Servings: 6-8
    Preparation Time: 20 minutes
    Cooking Time: none

THOUSAND ISLAND DRESSING

3/4 cup Kraft Fat-free Mayonnaise
3 tablespoons pickle relish
1 tablespoon minced bell pepper
1/2 cup tomato sauce
1 tablespoon minced onions
1 teaspoon lemon juice concentrate
1 package Nutra-Sweet or 2 teaspoons sugar (optional)

Blend ingredients with a fork or wire whisk. Cover and store in refrigerator. Best when used within 2 weeks.
    Servings: makes 1 1/2 cups
    Preparation Time: 15 minutes
    Cooking Time: none

Desserts

Lower in Calories - Fat-free - Cholesterol Free

FRUIT COBBLER

1 cup flour   1 cup fat-free soy milk
1 cup sugar   1 teaspoon baking powder

Mix together and pour into a 9"x13" non-stick baking dish. Sprinkle with butter buds and pour 1 quart fruit (any kind) with juice on top of batter. Bake at 350-375° for 45 minutes.
(To use unsweetened pie cherries, use 1/4 to 1/2 cups sugar dissolved in the cherries before adding to batter)
> Servings: 10-12
> Preparation Time: 5-10 minutes   Cooking Time: 40-45 minutes

---

BAKED RICE PUDDING

2 cups cooked brown rice   1 teaspoon vanilla
3 tablespoons honey   1 teaspoon cinnamon
1 1/2 cups fat-free soy milk   1 cup raisins
1 tablespoon quick-cooking tapioca   1 teaspoon nutmeg
Combine all ingredients. Pour into a casserole, cover, and bake at 325° for 45 minutes. May be served hot or cold.
> Servings: 4
> Preparation Time: 20 minutes   Cooking Time: 45 minutes

JELL-O FRUIT DELIGHT

1/2 angel food cake
1 large package Jell-O (same flavor as fruit)
1 16 oz. package frozen fruit
Tear angel food cake into bite size pieces. Prepare Jell-O as per directions using fruit juice as part of the liquid. Pour fruit and juice into Jell-O mixture, stir well. Refrigerate until syrupy, then into another bowl pour Jell-O and fruit mixture over cake pieces and refrigerate. This recipe is quick and easy to make. Your whole family will be delighted. Fat-free, Cholesterol Free.
> Servings: 8
> Preparation Time: 5-10 minutes   Cooking Time: none

BANANA GRAPE CUP

4 sliced bananas
1 cup orange juice
24 seedless green grapes
Dash nutmeg

Combine the sliced banana and the grapes in a dessert dish. Pour the orange juice over the fruit and sprinkle with nutmeg. Chill the fruits until they are ready to serve.

    Servings: 4
    Preparation Time: 5-10 minutes
    Cooking Time: none

CHERRY PIE

2 1/2 tablespoons tapioca
3 cups sweet cherries, frozen or fresh
1/8 teaspoon mace
1/4 teaspoon almond extract
1/4 cup Grape-Nut cereal
1/4 cup apple juice concentrate
2 tablespoons fruit juice
1/2 cup concentrated orange juice
1 pie crust (see recipe below)

Blend together the tapioca, mace, and orange juice; let stand for 15 minutes. Stir in the cherries and the almond extract. Pour into a nonstick pie pan lined with pie crust. Top with 1/4 cup of Grape-Nut cereal that has soaked 1 hour in the fruit juice. Bake in a preheated oven for about 40 minutes.

    Servings: makes 1 pie
    Preparation Time: 30 minutes
    Cooking Time: 40 minutes

PIE CRUST

1 cup Grape-Nut cereal, crushed
1/4 cup apple juice concentrate, undiluted

Combine Grape-Nuts and apple juice concentrate. Pat into a 9" pie pan.

CARROT PUDDING

2 cups cooked carrots
4 egg whites
1 15-oz. can crushed pineapple
1/2 cup raisins
1/4 cup honey
5 slices whole wheat bread
2 tablespoons grated orange rind
1 teaspoon cinnamon
1/4 teaspoon allspice
1/4 teaspoon nutmeg

Steam carrots until tender. Meanwhile, beat egg whites until stiff peaks form. Put the pineapple in a blender with the cooked carrots; puree. Tear the bread into tiny pieces; put the carrot-pineapple puree over the bread and mix lightly. Add orange rind, raisins, honey, and spices. Mix lightly. Add beaten egg whites and fold in. Bake in 8" x 10" nonstick pan at 350° for 45 minutes, or until knife in center comes out clean and top is brown.

Servings: 6
Preparation Time: 20 minutes
Cooking Time: 45 minutes

BANANA STRAWBERRY FREEZE

8 frozen bananas, sliced
1 cup frozen strawberries, unsweetened
1 cup cold water

Place sliced bananas into blender. Blend, adding a little water at a time. Use only enough water to give the consistency of ice cream. Use less water if using a food processor. Break up frozen strawberries and blend into banana mixture until smooth. Serve immediately. To freeze bananas, peel, slice and wrap in plastic wrap or baggie, and freeze for about 12 hours.

Servings: 4
Preparation Time: 10 minutes

BLUEBERRY UPSIDE DOWN CAKE

1/4 cup packed brown sugar
2 tablespoons light corn syrup
1 tablespoon lemon juice
1 cup fresh or frozen blueberries
WHITE CAKE batter (recipe follows)

Lightly spray a 9 inch round non-stick cake pan with cooking spray. Add brown sugar, corn syrup and lemon juice; stir to combine. Place pan in a 350° oven 3 minutes. Remove. Add blueberries. Prepare WHITE CAKE batter. Carefully spoon batter over blueberries, smoothing top. Bake 35 to 40 minutes or until toothpick inserted in center comes out clean. (Do not over bake.) Immediately run spatula around edge of pan and invert cake onto serving plate. Other fruits can be used for variety.

This is a delectable dessert, low in calories, Fat-free, and Cholesterol Free.

    Servings: 12
    Preparation Time: 25 minutes
    Cooking Time: 35-40 minutes

WHITE CAKE

1 cup flour
2/3 cup sugar
2 teaspoons baking powder
1/3 cup cornstarch
1/2 teaspoon salt (optional)

3 teaspoons ENER-G egg
    replacer or 2 egg whites
2/3 cup non-fat soy milk
1/3 cup light corn syrup
1 teaspoon vanilla

In a large bowl combine flour, sugar, baking powder, corn starch, and salt. In medium bowl, using fork or wire whisk mix egg replacer or egg whites, milk, corn syrup and vanilla. Add to flour mixture; stir until smooth. Pour into a 9"x9" non-stick baking pan. Bake in 350° oven 20 to 25 minutes or until toothpick inserted in center comes out clean. Cool in pan on wire rack.

This cake is light as a feather. Serve with fresh or frozen fruit as a frosting- Raspberries are especially delicious. Fat-free, Cholesterol Free.

    Servings: 16
    Preparation Time: 20 minutes
    Cooking Time: 20-25 minutes

CHOCOLATE CAKE

1 1/4 cup flour
1 cup sugar
1/3 cup carob powder
(carob powder is nearly fat-free)
1/4 cup corn syrup
1/2 teaspoon baking soda

1/2 teaspoon salt (optional)
6 teaspoons egg replacer mixed
  with 8 tablespoons water or
  4 egg whites
1 cup water
1/2 cup light or dark corn syrup

Preheat oven to 350°. Use a 9" square non-stick baking . In large bowl combine dry ingredients until well mixed. In medium bowl mix egg replacer or egg whites, water and corn syrup. Stir into dry ingredients until smooth. Pour into prepared pan. Bake 30 minutes or until cake springs back when lightly touched. Cool on wire rack 10 minutes.
Low in calories, Fat-Free, Cholesterol Free.
  Servings: 16
  Preparation Time: 20 minutes
  Cooking Time: 30 minutes

SPICE CAKE

1 cup whole wheat flour
2 teaspoons baking powder
2/3 cup brown sugar
1/3 cup corn starch
1/2 teaspoon cinnamon
1/8 teaspoon ground ginger
1/2 teaspoon salt (optional)

1/8 teaspoon nutmeg
1/3 cup dark corn syrup
2/3 cup non-fat soy milk
3 teaspoons ENER-G egg
  replacer or 2 egg whites
1 teaspoon vanilla

In a large bowl combine flour, brown sugar, corn starch, baking powder, cinnamon, ginger and nutmeg. In a medium bowl, using a fork or wire whisk, mix egg replacer or egg whites, milk, corn syrup and vanilla. Add to flour mixture; stir until smooth. Pour into a 9"x9" non-stick pan. Bake in 350° oven 25 to 30 minutes or until toothpick comes out clean. Cool in pan on wire rack. Serve with applesauce for an old-fashioned treat.
Only 100 calories per serving, Fat-Free, Cholesterol Free.
  Servings: 16
  Preparation Time: 20 minutes
  Cooking Time: 25-30 minutes

NO-FAT CARROT CAKE

2 cups whole wheat flour
3/4 teaspoon allspice
1 1/2 cups unsweetened applesauce
1 3/4 teaspoons cinnamon
3/4 cup honey
1/2 teaspoon nutmeg
3 egg whites or 4 teaspoons of egg replacer mixed in 7 teaspoons of water
3 cups grated carrots
1/4 teaspoon cloves
1 1/4 teaspoons baking soda
2 teaspoons baking powder
1 8-oz. can crushed pineapple
1/2 cup raisins

Mix dry ingredients together. Mix moist ingredients together. Add flour mixture to moist ingredients. Stir gently until mixed. Add carrots, pineapple, and raisins. Stir well. Pour mixture into a nonstick 13 x 9 x 2 pan. Bake at 350° for 60 minutes.
Low in calories, no cholesterol, no fat.
    Servings: 10
    Preparation Time: 25 minutes
    Cooking Time: 1 hour

ROCKY MOUNTAIN FROSTING

1 cup sugar
1 teaspoon cream of tartar
1/2 cup water
2 egg whites
1 tsp. vanilla

Cook sugar, cream of tartar, and water together until hard ball forms when dropped in water. Meanwhile beat egg whites until stiff. Beat hot syrup into egg whites until stiff peaks form again. Add vanilla
    Preparation Time: 15 minutes

OATMEAL-BANANA COOKIES

Sift Together:

1 cup whole wheat flour
1/2 teaspoon baking soda
1/2 teaspoon baking powder
1/4 teaspoon cream of tartar
1 teaspoon cinnamon
1 teaspoon vanilla
1/2 cup apple juice concentrate

Add to sifted ingredients:

2 mashed ripe bananas
3 tablespoons applesauce
1 cup oatmeal
1/3 cup raisins*
1/2 cup chopped dates
2 tablespoons honey

Drop by teaspoons on non-stick cookie sheet. Bake 10 to 15 minutes in 350°
oven.
*1/2 cup of carob chips can be substituted for raisins.
NOTE: Carob contains less than 9 percent fat
      Servings: 24 cookies
      Preparation Time: 15 minutes
      Cooking Time: 10-15 minutes

BROWNIE OAT COOKIES

2/3 cup whole wheat flour
2/3 cup sugar
1 cup quick oats
1/8 cup carob powder
1 teaspoon baking powder
3 teaspoons ENER-G egg replacer
 or 2 egg whites

1/3 cup dark corn syrup
1 teaspoon vanilla
1/4 teaspoon salt (optional)

In a large bowl combine flour, sugar, oats, carob powder, baking powder and
salt. Add egg replacer or egg whites, corn syrup and vanilla; stir just until
dry ingredients are moistened. Drop by teaspoonfuls onto non-stick cookie
sheets. Bake in 350° oven 10 minutes or until set. Cool 5 minutes on cookie
sheets. Remove; cool on wire rack.
No fat, no cholesterol, limited calories.
      Servings: 24 cookies
      Preparation Time: 15 minutes
      Cooking Time: 10 minutes

BAKED FRUIT SALAD SUPREME

1 16-oz. can pineapple chunks (in own juice, drained with juice reserved)
1 tablespoon tapioca
1 fresh apple, diced
1 orange, peeled and diced
4 tablespoons frozen pineapple juice concentrate
2 egg whites
1/8 teaspoon cream of tartar
1/2 teaspoon vanilla
2 teaspoons Sucrose

Bring reserved pineapple juice and tapioca to a boil until thickened. Combine the apple, pineapple, orange, and frozen pineapple juice concentrate. Mix well to coat fruits with the thickened juice. Spoon fruit into 4 individual souffle baking dishes. Beat egg whites until soft peaks form. Add the cream of tartar and Sucrose and continue beating until stiff peaks form. Add vanilla. Swirl the egg whites to top of the fruit salad, heaping it thick and spreading it to edges of dishes. Place in pre-heated 450° oven for 4 to 5 minutes until meringue is lightly browned.

Servings: 4
Preparation Time: 20 minutes
Cooking Time: 5 minutes

RASPBERRY FROZEN DESSERT

1 1/2 cups canned unsweetened crushed pineapple with juice
3 frozen bananas
3 cups frozen raspberries (1 16-oz. bag, low sugar)

To freeze bananas, peel, cut up, and freeze in a plastic bag for at least 12 hours. Place the bananas, pineapple and juice in the blender. Add the frozen raspberries a little at a time, blending well. Place 1/2 cup of mixture into each of 8 dessert dishes and freeze for 15-30 minutes. If ingredients are frozen for a longer period of time, remove from freezer a short while before serving.

Servings: 8
Preparation Time: 10 minutes
Cooking Time: none (requires 15-30 minutes freezing time)

SPICE RAISIN COOKIES

2/3 cup whole wheat flour   1/3 cup dark corn syrup
2/3 cup sugar   1/4 teaspoon cinnamon
1 cup quick oatmeal   dash nutmeg
1 teaspoon baking powder   dash ginger
1/4 teaspoon salt (optional)   1/8 cup raisins
3 teaspoons ENER-G egg replacer   1 teaspoon vanilla
  or 2 egg whites

In a large bowl combine flour, sugar, oats, baking powder and salt. Add egg replacer or egg whites, corn syrup and vanilla; stir just until dry ingredients are moistened. Drop by teaspoonfuls onto non-stick cookie sheets. Bake in 350° oven 10 minutes or until set. Cool 5 minutes on cookie sheet. Remove; cool on wire rack.

    Servings: about 2 dozen cookies
    Preparation Time: 15 minutes
    Cooking Time: 10-15 minutes

APPLE PIE

1 cup Grape-Nuts cereal, crushed
1/4 cup apple juice concentrate
1 can apples, packed in water
1/2 cup apple juice concentrate
1 tablespoon lemon juice
1 1/2 teaspoons apple pie spice, or 1/2 teaspoon nutmeg,
  1/4 teaspoon allspice and 1 teaspoon cinnamon
1 tablespoon tapioca
2 tablespoons honey

For pie crust combine Grape-Nuts and 1/4 cup apple juice concentrate. Pat into a 9-inch pie pan. Place apples, concentrate, and tapioca in a saucepan; bring to a boil. Boil about 2 minutes. Stir in remaining ingredients. Pour into Grape-Nuts crust. Sprinkle a few crushed Grape-Nuts over top. Cover with foil and bake 1/2 hour at 350°.

    Servings: 6
    Preparation Time: 20 minutes
    Cooking Time: 30 minutes

JAN'S MEXICAN FRUIT CAKE

2 cups flour
2 cups sugar
2 teaspoons baking soda
4 teaspoons egg replacer or 3 egg whites
1 20-oz. can crushed pineapple with juice
1 8 oz. can crushed pineapple without juice

Mix ingredients together and pour into 9 x 13 non-stick pan. Bake at 350°
for 40-45 minutes.
    Servings: 12
    Preparation Time: 5 minutes
    Cooking Time: 45 minutes

BAKED APPLES

4 apples, peeled
Apple pie spice
4 tablespoons undiluted frozen apple juice concentrate, thawed
4 teaspoons seedless raisins

Core apples; sprinkle apple pie spice into the core cavity. Fill each core with
1 tablespoon apple juice and 1 teaspoon raisins. Place apples in a small baking dish. Bake in a 350° oven for 1 hour or until the apples are fork tender.
    Servings: 4
    Preparation Time:15-20 minutes
    Cooking Time: 1 hour

Breakfast

EASY PANCAKES

1 1/2 cups whole wheat flour   1 3/4 teaspoons baking powder
1 3/4 cups water   1/4 teaspoon apple pie spice

Mix dry ingredients, then add water and mix well. Spoon onto non-stick griddle or pan. Turn when bubbles appear.
   Servings: 8-10 pancakes

FROZEN HASH-BROWN POTATOES

1 package frozen hash-brown potatoes (choose a brand with no added oil)
1/2 cup chopped onion
1/8 teaspoon Mrs. Dash
Pepper to taste

Cook in a nonstick skillet over medium heat for 15 minutes; turn and cook for 10 minutes on other side, until browned. Garnish with ketchup or other sauce (no-oil).
   Servings: 1 (eat all you want)
   Preparation Time: 1 minute
   Cooking Time: 25 minutes

BANANA-APPLESAUCE PANCAKES

1 cup whole wheat flour   2 tablespoons unsweetened
1 medium banana   applesauce
1 1/2 teaspoons baking powder   1 teaspoon honey
1 1/4 cup non-fat soy milk or apple juice   1/2 teaspoon vanilla

Mix flour and baking powder together. Mix liquid with applesauce and honey. Add to dry ingredients and stir until just moistened. Fold in chopped banana. Spoon batter onto a medium-heat, nonstick griddle. Turn cakes when bubbles appear. These pancakes are great with applesauce and cinnamon on them.
   Servings: makes 12 pancakes
   Preparation Time: 10 minutes
   Cooking Time: 15 minutes

TRIPLE-MIX CEREAL

5 cups Wheatena
5 cups oatmeal
5 cups oat bran

Mix dry ingredients in a large container; store covered. To make 2 quarts of cooked cereal: Boil 2 quarts of water in a 3-quart pan. Stir into boiling water 2 cups of dry mix. Turn heat to medium or medium low; cook for 30 minutes or longer. Add water as needed. For variety, stir in a little unsweetened applesauce or sprinkle on cinnamon or apple pie spice. If you need milk, try diluted fat-free soy milk or fat-free rice milk.

  Servings: 1 cup dry mix makes
    1 quart cereal

OTHER HOT CEREALS

Generally, cook all whole-grain hot cereals in 3 parts water to 1 part cereal, using more or less water as desired. For a variety of tastes, add a little honey, cinnamon, bananas, prunes, raisins, dates, or other dried fruit. (Fat-free rice milk or fat-free soy milk, vanilla or plain, are great on cereals)

Seven-grain cereal   Oatmeal
Millet
If you enjoy more of a porridge consistency, blend to a cornmeal texture before cooking. This will cut the cooking time in half. Raisins or other dried fruit go well with millet.

Cornmeal   Buckwheat groats
Groats are pre-toasted and cook quickly compared to other whole grains. They have a uniquely strong flavor.

Wheatena   Roman Meal
Zoom   Whole-grain wheat, oats, or rye
Whole grains need a long cooking time. Soak them overnight in water. Cook in 3 parts water to 1 part cereal until they are tender enough to eat. They can be very chewy and take a long time to eat. To cut the eating time, place in a blender and grind up the grain after cooking. This makes an old-time porridge mixture.

FRENCH TOAST

2 slices of whole-grain bread or pita bread
1 teaspoon egg-replacer or 2 egg whites
1/4 teaspoon vanilla
1 teaspoon cinnamon
1/4 cup non-fat soy milk
1/4 cup unsweetened thawed frozen orange juice

Soak the bread in a blended mixture of all other ingredients. Cook on a non-stick griddle, or bake in the oven on a nonstick pan for 10 minutes on each side. Serve hot.
   Servings: 1

PUMPKIN BRAN MUFFINS

1 1/2 cups whole wheat flour
2 teaspoons baking powder
1/2 teaspoon baking soda
1/2 teaspoon salt (optional)
1 teaspoon cinnamon
3 teaspoons ENER-G egg replacer or 2 egg whites
1 cup canned pumpkin
1 cup wheat bran
3/4 cup fat-free soy milk
1/2 cup Karo corn syrup
1 teaspoon vanilla

In medium bowl combine flour, baking powder, baking soda, salt and cinnamon. In a large bowl, using a fork or wire whisk, beat egg whites lightly or use 3 teaspoons of egg replacer mixed thoroughly with 4 tablespoons water. Stir in pumpkin, wheat bran, vanilla, milk and corn syrup. Add flour mixture; stir until well blended. Spoon into non-stick muffin cups. Bake in 400° oven 18 to 20 minutes or until lightly browned and firm to touch. Cool in pan 5 minutes. Remove; cool on wire rack. Fat-free, Cholesterol Free, High Fiber. These can be frozen for future use.
   Servings: 12 muffins
   Preparation Time: 25 minutes
   Cooking Time: 20 minutes

BANANA MUFFINS

1 1/2 cups whole wheat flour
1/4 cup wheat bran
2 teaspoons baking powder
1/2 teaspoon baking soda
1/2 teaspoon salt (optional)
1 teaspoon vanilla

1/2 teaspoon cinnamon
3 teaspoons egg replacer or
  2 egg whites
2 large, ripe bananas, mashed
2/3 cup non-fat soy milk
1/3 cup Karo corn syrup

Use 12 (2 1/2 inch) non-stick muffin cups. In medium bowl combine all dry ingredients. In a large bowl beat egg whites lightly, or use 3 teaspoons of ENER-G egg replacer mixed thoroughly with 4 tablespoons water. Stir in mashed bananas, milk and corn syrup. Add flour mixture; stir until well blended. Spoon into prepared muffin cups. Bake in 400° oven 22 to 25 minutes or until firm to touch. Cool in pan 5 minutes. Remove: cool on wire rack. Fat-free, Cholesterol Free, High Fiber and Low in calories. Good source of complex carbohydrate.

   Servings: 12 muffins
   Preparation Time: 20 minutes
   Cooking Time: 25 minutes

BREAKFAST MUFFINS

2 cups whole wheat flour
2 teaspoons baking powder
1/2 teaspoon baking soda
1/4 cup corn syrup
1 1/2 cups non-fat soy milk
2 teaspoons egg replacer mixed with 4 tablespoons water
2 tablespoons apple sauce

Combine dry ingredients. Combine liquid ingredients. Fold dry and liquid ingredients together, until just moistened. Spoon into nonstick muffin pans. Bake at 400° for 18 to 20 minutes until lightly browned and firm to the touch. For a different taste use 1 cup cornmeal in place of 1 cup flour. Try 1/2 cup raisins; 1/2 teaspoon cinnamon or 1/4 teaspoon nutmeg, ginger, or allspice for variety.

   Servings: makes 12 muffins
   Preparation Time: 10 minutes
   Cooking Time: 18-20 minutes

WHOLE-KERNEL WHEAT WAFFLES

1 cup whole wheat kernels
1 1/2 cups non-fat soy milk
2 egg whites or 3 teaspoons egg replacer (ENER-G)
1/2 teaspoon vanilla
4 teaspoons baking powder
1 tablespoon honey

Place wheat kernels and milk in blender. Blend until smooth. Add egg whites, honey, and baking powder. Blend all ingredients. Let batter rest 10 minutes. Ladle onto preheated nonstick waffle iron. (Use about 1 cup of batter for a 4 section waffle.) Serve with all-fruit jam, honey, or maple syrup. For pancakes, use only 1 egg white or 1 teaspoon egg replacer.

> Servings: makes 2 waffles
> Preparation Time: 15 minutes
> Cooking Time: 25 minutes

VARIOUS COLD CEREALS

Shredded Wheat (spoon-size or regular)
Use spoon-size Shredded Wheat as a convenient snack anywhere, any time.
Grape-Nuts
Carry a little plastic sack of Grape-Nuts with you for snacks. It contains
   some salt, but makes a handy, healthful snack.
Granola (with no added fats)
Puffed Wheat (Arrowhead Mills)
Puffed Corn (Arrowhead Mills)
Puffed Rice (Arrowhead Mills)
Oat Bran O's (Health Valley Foods)
Skinner's Raisin Bran (US Mills)
100 Percent Natural Bran Cereal (Health Valley Foods)

Breads

100% WHOLE WHEAT BREAD

2 1/2 teaspoons or 1 pkg. dry yeast
3 cups whole wheat flour
1/4 cup gluten flour
1/8 cup cracked wheat
1/2 to 1 teaspoon salt (optional)
1 1/4 cup hot water (125° - 130°)
2 tablespoon molasses or honey
3 teaspoons ENER-G egg replacer mixed thoroughly
  with 4 tablespoons water or 2 egg whites

In the order listed, put all ingredients in bread machine pan. Select white bread and push to start. For Cinnamon Raisin Bread: at the beep sound in the second mixing, add 1 1/2 tablespoons cinnamon and 3/4 cup raisins.

NOTE: For 100% Whole Wheat No-Fat Dinner Rolls: Turn BREAD MA-CHINE off after "beep, beep, beep." Make dough into 18 equal balls, place in non-stick muffin tins. Let rise 2 hours or until doubles in size. Bake at 400° for about 12 to 15 minutes. Balls of dough can be frozen for future use. Let rise for 3 or 4 hours before baking.
    Preparation Time: 5 minutes using BREAD MACHINE

DIANE'S WHOLE WHEAT BANANA BREAD

1 cup unsweetened applesauce   1 teaspoon salt (optional)
6 medium bananas   2 teaspoons baking soda
1 1/2 cups honey   4 cups whole wheat flour
2 egg whites or 3 teaspoons egg replacer (ENER-G brand)

Combine applesauce, honey, and slightly beaten egg whites or egg replacer. When thoroughly mixed, add mashed bananas and remaining ingredients. Pour into nonstick loaf pans. Bake at 325° for 1 hour and 10 minutes.
    Servings: makes 2 loaves
    Preparation Time: 30 minutes
    Cooking Time: 70 minutes

DOROTHY'S HONEY WHOLE WHEAT BREAD

4 cups whole wheat flour   2 packages dry yeast
3 cups water   3/4 cup wheat bran or oat bran
1/2 cup non-fat soy milk   1 teaspoon salt (optional)
1/2 cup honey   4 cups bread flour
1/4 cup bulgur wheat (soaked in hot water)

Combine in a large bowl 4 cups whole wheat flour, 1 teaspoon salt, and 2 packages dry yeast. In a saucepan combine 3 cups water, 1/2 cup nonfat soy milk, 1/2 cup honey; heat until 105° to 115°. Pour liquid over flour mixture. Blend at low speed 1 minute, medium speed 2 minutes. By hand, stir in 1 cup whole wheat flour, 3/4 cup wheat or oat bran cereal, 1/4 cup bulgur wheat, and 4 cups bread flour. Knead on floured surface about 5 minutes. Place dough in non-stick bowl; cover and let rise 45 to 60 minutes until doubled. Punch down, divide in half, knead, and shape into loaves. Put in two 9 x 5 non-stick loaf pans (sprinkle pans with cornmeal to make removing easier). Cover and let rise 30 to 45 minutes until doubled. Bake at 350° for 40-45 minutes. Remove from pans and cool on wire racks.
  Servings: makes 2 loaves
  Preparation Time: 45 minutes
  Cooking Time: 45 minutes
  Rising Time: 1 1/2 hours

SWEET POTATO AND RAISIN BREAD

1 package dry yeast, 2 1/2 tablespoons   3 teaspoons egg replacer or
2 cups flour   2 egg whites
1 cup whole wheat flour   1 cup mashed sweet potatoes
1/4 cup light brown sugar   1 tablespoon corn syrup
1 teaspoon salt (optional)   1/2 cup warm water (115°)

Place all ingredients in BREAD MACHINE in order listed. Select white bread and push "Start". At the sound of the "Beep, beep, beep in the second mixing, add 2/3 cup raisins.

NOTE: Rapid-Rise yeast seems to work better at high altitudes. When using Rapid-Rise yeast use hotter water (125° to 130°).
  Preparation Time: 5 minutes using BREAD MACHINE.

OAT BRAN MUFFINS

2 cups whole wheat flour
2 cups mashed bananas (3 or 4 bananas)
1 cup oat bran
4 teaspoons baking powder
3/4 cup apple juice
1 1/2 teaspoons cinnamon
1/2 cup raisins
1 egg white or 1 teaspoon egg replacer

Lightly oil nonstick muffin tins. Sift dry ingredients together; add bananas, raisins, and apple juice. Stir until just mixed. Fill muffin tins and bake at 350° for 30 minutes.

Servings: makes 18 muffins
Preparation Time: 15 minutes
Cooking Time: 30 minutes

GOOD CORN BREAD

1 cup cornmeal
1 cup non-fat soy milk
1 cup flour
4 teaspoons baking powder
1/2 cup frozen corn
1/2 teaspoon salt (optional)
4 oz. green chilies, diced and/or 4 oz. jalapeno chilies
1 egg white or 2 teaspoons egg replacer

Mix dry ingredients together. Mix moist ingredients together along with diced chilies and frozen corn. Add dry ingredients to wet ingredients. Mix. Place in a non-stick 8-inch baking pan. (Sprinkle pans with cornmeal to make removing easier). Bake at 425° oven for 25 to 30 minutes.

Servings: 4
Preparation Time: 15 minutes
Cooking Time: 25 minutes

Vegetables and Side Dishes

ASPARAGUS DELIGHT

Fresh or frozen asparagus
Homemade whole wheat croutons (Mrs. Dash no-salt herb seasoning and
dill weed)

Steam asparagus 8 to 10 minutes or until tender. Cut up whole wheat bread
slices into small squares. Place on a nonstick cookie sheet. Sprinkle a little
Mrs. Dash and dill weed over bread cubes. Toast in a 275° oven until dried
out. Place the toasted bread cubes over the hot asparagus before serving.
> Servings: 4
> Preparation Time: 10 minutes
> Cooking Time: 8-10 minutes

SPICED BEETS

1 pound beets   1/8 teaspoon cloves
1/4 teaspoon Mrs. Dash   1/4 teaspoon allspice

Cook whole beets for 40 minutes or until tender. Peel. Combine the herbs
and spices and sprinkle over each serving of beets.
> Servings: 4
> Preparation Time: 5 minutes
> Cooking Time: 40 minutes

BROCCOLI

2 heads broccoli (trim off most of stem)
Pepper to taste
1/4 teaspoon Mrs. Dash

Cook (steam) broccoli in a small amount of water 15 minutes or until tender.
Sprinkle with Mrs. Dash and pepper during last 2 minutes of cooking time.
Serve hot.
> Servings: 4
> Preparation Time: 5 minutes
> Cooking Time: 15 minutes

CABBAGE SPECIAL

4 cups shredded cabbage	1 tablespoon honey
3 onions, diced	2 cooking apples, diced
1/4 cup apple juice	1/4 teaspoon Mrs. Dash
1 lemon, juiced, or	1/4 cup raisins
1 tablespoon lemon juice	

Place all ingredients in a saucepan and bring to a boil Lower heat to medium-low and simmer for about 10 minutes, or until barely tender but still crisp. Do not overcook.

Servings: 4-6
Preparation Time: 15 minutes
Cooking Time: 10 minutes

BAKED POTATOES

Prepare potatoes by scrubbing; bake at 400° for 1 to 1 1/2 hours. Size of potatoes determines cooking time. Store unused potatoes in refrigerator. A little pepper will be sufficient seasoning for many people. You can also try a little Mrs. Dash no-salt seasoning, chunky vegetables, pea soup, onion soup, nonfat salad dressings, oriental vegetables, or ketchup.

Servings: variable
Preparation Time: 3 minutes
Cooking Time: 1 - 1 1/2 hours
    (Microwave baked potatoes: 1 in 6 minutes; 2 in 9 minutes)

MASHED POTATOES

4 or 5 medium potatoes, cut into chunks
Place potatoes in a large saucepan; add water to cover. Bring to a boil. Cover and cook over medium heat about 20 minutes or until tender. Drain off some of the liquid and keep for future soups or gravies. Whip by hand or with an electric mixer until smooth. For variety, add 2 tablespoons of fat-free soy milk to make it creamier. A little Mrs. Dash and black pepper spices up mashed potatoes. Use your favorite spices, but no fats. For variety in color and flavor, boil 3 medium carrots or one large stalk of broccoli, cut into chunks, along with your potatoes. Add 10 minutes or more to your cooking time. Mash carrots or broccoli with the potatoes.

Servings: 4
Preparation Time: 10 minutes   Cooking Time: 20 minutes

POTATOES AND CABBAGE

4 unpeeled chunked potatoes
2 carrots, sliced
1 onion, chopped
1/4 teaspoon Mrs. Dash
2 cups chopped cabbage
1/8 teaspoon fennel (optional)
2 stalks sliced celery
1/8 teaspoon black pepper

Place all vegetables in a 3-quart saucepan and cover with water. Bring to a boil, turn to medium heat. Cover and steam for 15 minutes. Add spices and cook 5 minutes more or until tender.

    Servings: 4-6
    Preparation Time: 20 minutes
    Cooking Time: 20 minutes

CAULIFLOWER

Place cauliflower in saucepan; add enough water to steam for 7-10 minutes without burning. Sprinkle with Mrs. Dash, pepper, and paprika for flavor and color.

    Servings: variable
    Preparation Time: 5 minutes
    Cooking Time: 7-10 minutes

CORN ON THE COB

Shuck the corn. Place 3 inches or more water in a large pot. Bring water to a boil. Place ears of corn in the water. Cook for 5 to 10 minutes if corn is young; more mature corn needs 5 minutes or more extra cooking. Don't over-cook. Microwave instructions: Place corn in plastic bag. Cook 1 ear 4 minutes; 2 ears 7 minutes; 3 ears 10 minutes; 4 ears 13 minutes. Corn can be microwaved with husks on.

    Servings: variable
    Preparation Time: 10 minutes
    Cooking Time: 5-10 minutes

SPINACH

1 box frozen spinach   Dash of pepper
Dash of Mrs. Dash   Vinegar, lemon juice (optional)

Place 1/4 inch water in saucepan. Bring to a boil; add spinach and steam 5 minutes, or until tender. Don't overcook. Flavor with Mrs. Dash, pepper, and lemon juice or vinegar.

   Servings: 2
   Preparation Time: 3 minutes
   Cooking Time: 5 minutes

SPINACH COMBO

2 bunches fresh spinach or 2 boxes frozen spinach
1/2 teaspoon Mrs. Dash   2 unpeeled potatoes, chunked
2 medium tomatoes, chopped   Dash of pepper

Place 2 inches of water in a large pot with the spinach. Steam until spinach starts to wilt. Add the tomatoes and potatoes. Continue cooking until potatoes are tender. Add Mrs. Dash and pepper during the last 5 minutes of cooking.

   Servings: 4
   Preparation Time: 5 minutes
   Cooking Time: 15 minutes

OKRA

2 cups frozen cut okra   1 medium onion, chopped
1 cup tomato juice, salted or unsalted   1/4 teaspoon oregano
1/4 teaspoon garlic powder   1/4 teaspoon Mrs. Dash
Dash of cayenne pepper
2 slices whole wheat bread made into crumbs
Combine all ingredients except bread crumbs. Place in a nonstick baking dish and sprinkle with bread crumbs. Bake in a preheated 350° oven for 45 minutes.

   Servings: 4
   Preparation Time: 5 minutes
   Cooking Time: 45 minutes

BROWN RICE

1 cup brown rice
1/4 teaspoon Mrs. Dash
2 1/2 cups water

1/8 teaspoon pepper
1/4 teaspoon onion powder
Dash of cayenne pepper

Place rice in a baking dish with a tight-fitting lid. Cover rice with water. Season with Mrs. Dash, onion powder, pepper, and cayenne. Bake in a 350° oven for 1 hour.
> Servings: 4
> Preparation Time: 5 minutes
> Cooking Time: 1 hour

BREADED MUSHROOMS DELUXE

1 pound fresh mushrooms, sliced
5 slices whole wheat bread, crumbled

4 egg whites, beaten
2 teaspoons Mrs. Dash

Wash mushrooms. Dip the sliced mushrooms into the beaten egg whites and place on a non-stick cookie sheet. Combine Mrs. Dash seasoning with the bread crumbs; sprinkle over the mushrooms. Bake in 350° oven for 20 minutes or until tender and crisp.
> Servings: 6-8
> Preparation Time: 15 minutes
> Cooking Time: 20 minutes

WINTER SQUASH

1 butternut, banana, or acorn squash
1/2 teaspoon cinnamon
1 tablespoon honey
1/2 teaspoon nutmeg

Cut squash in half and remove seeds. Place in an open baking pan with the inside of squash face up. Brush with honey, cinnamon, and nutmeg mixture. Bake at 300° for 1 hour.
> Servings: 4
> Preparation Time: 5 minutes
> Cooking Time: 1 hour

HASH BROWN POTATOES

Regular size frozen Bel-Air Hash Brown Potatoes (or other no-oil brand)
1 onion, chopped
1/4 teaspoon pepper
1/4 teaspoon Mrs. Dash

Defrost potatoes in microwave oven for 3 or 4 minutes. (If you don't have a microwave, defrost in skillet as it cooks.) Heat nonstick skillet. Add onions and 2 or 3 tablespoons of water. Saute for 2 minutes. Add hash brown potatoes and spices. Turn heat to medium high and cook for 20-25 minutes, or until browned to your liking. Turn occasionally with a non-metal spatula. Serve with ketchup or barbecue sauce.
      Servings: 2-4
      Preparation Time: 10 minutes
      Cooking Time: 20-25 minutes

OVEN FRIED POTATOES

Wash and dry, but do not peel, 4 potatoes. Drop into a pot of boiling water, lower heat to simmer, and cook until barely tender. Remove from the pot and refrigerate. Alternate method-Microwave 4 potatoes for 15 minutes; don't overcook. Refrigerate. When potatoes are cool, peel them carefully and slice length-wise as for french fries. Spread the potatoes on a nonstick baking sheet and season with onion powder, garlic powder, paprika, black pepper, and/or chili powder. Brown in a 400° oven and turn with a spatula to brown the other side. Potatoes will be crispy.
      Servings: 4
      Preparation Time: 10 minutes
      Cooking Time: 20-25 minutes

SEASONED CORN

3 cups frozen corn
1 4-oz. can green chiles, chopped
1 2-oz. jar pimientos

Combine and cook for about 5 minutes. Do not overcook.
      Servings: 4-6
      Preparation Time: 5 minutes
      Cooking Time: 5 minutes

HERBED CARROTS

4 cups sliced carrots
1/2 cup minced onion
2 tablespoons rice vinegar
1 teaspoon basil
2 cloves garlic
Dash salt (at table)

Blanch carrots in boiling water for 2 minutes. (To blanch, place carrots in boiling water; let water come back to a boil for 2 minutes. Plunge immediately into cold water to stop the cooking.) Drain; add the herbs, vinegar, and onion to the carrots. Note: Recipe can be used with any herb of your choice. Experiment!
  Servings: 4-6
  Preparation Time: 10 minutes
  Cooking Time: 5 minutes

BULGUR WITH VEGETABLES

2 cups bulgur wheat
1 cup carrots, sliced
1 teaspoon tarragon
4 green onions, sliced
1 cup broccoli, sliced
2 cloves garlic, minced
1 teaspoon basil
2 tablespoons rice vinegar

Place bulgur in a large microwave dish. Cover with water and cook in microwave for 8-10 minutes, or until water is absorbed. Blanch the carrots and broccoli. Combine bulgur and the vegetables; mix in the garlic, onions, vinegar, and spices. Chill before serving.
  Servings: 4-6
  Preparation Time: 15 minutes
  Cooking Time: 10-15 minutes

This and That

APPLE BUTTER

1 quart unsweetened applesauce   1 3/4 teaspoons cinnamon
1/4 teaspoon ground cloves   1/2 teaspoon allspice

Combine all ingredients in a saucepan and cook over medium-low heat for 1 hour. This apple butter can be used as a spread on bread, toast, pancakes, waffles, and many other ways in place of butter, margarine, peanut butter, and other spreads. It contains less than 1 percent fat and no cholesterol.

    Servings: variable
    Preparation Time: 5 minutes
    Cooking Time: 1 hour

HOT CINNAMON APPLESAUCE

1 cup unsweetened applesauce
1/2 teaspoon cinnamon

Heat applesauce over medium heat on stove, or heat in microwave oven. Add 1/2 teaspoon cinnamon. Use as a topping for whole wheat waffles or pancakes, toast, bread, and bagels. Contains less than 1 percent fat and no cholesterol.

    Servings: variable
    Preparation Time: 2 minutes
    Cooking Time: none

STRAWBERRY BREAKFAST SPREAD

1 teaspoon unflavored gelatin   4 teaspoons Sucrose
1/4 cup orange juice   1 tablespoon orange peel slivers
1/4 teaspoon coriander
1 cup mashed or pureed fresh or frozen unsweetened strawberries

In a small saucepan, sprinkle gelatin over orange juice. Let stand 1 minute. Heat over low heat until gelatin is dissolved and mixture comes to a boil. Remove from heat and stir into strawberries. Add remaining ingredients and stir to blend. Refrigerate until firm, 3 to 4 hours. Best when used within 1 week.

    Servings: makes 1 cup
    Preparation Time: 10 minutes
    Cooking Time: 15 minutes

VEGETABLE DIP

1 pint Kraft Fat-free Mayonnaise
2 teaspoons Beau Monde
2 teaspoons dill weed
2 teaspoons minced onion
2 teaspoons parsley flakes

Add all spices to Mayo. Use as a dip or serve over baked potatoes.
    Servings: variable
    Preparation Time: 5-10 minutes
    Cooking Time: none

BEAN DIP

2 cups cooked beans, mashed or canned Fat-free Refried Beans
1/8 teaspoon Tabasco sauce
1/2 teaspoon Extra Spicy Mrs. Dash
1/2 teaspoon chili powder
1/2 teaspoon salt (optional)
1/4 cup green chilies
1/4 teaspoon seasoned pepper

Mix all ingredients well. Use this in place of commercial bean dips. Contains only 3 percent fat and no cholesterol, while many commercial bean dips contain a high percentage of animal lard, cholesterol, and salt.
    Servings: variable
    Preparation Time: 5-10 minutes
    Cooking Time: none

CORN TORTILLA CHIPS

Packaged corn and lime tortillas; available in packages of 1 or 3 dozen.
Cut tortillas in eighths. Put on a nonstick cookie sheet and bake about 30 minutes at 350°, stirring once. Contain no cholesterol, no salt, and only about 8 percent fat, while some commercial corn chips contain considerable salt and up to 80 grams of fat (720 calories) for an 8 oz. bag.
    Servings: variable
    Preparation Time: 10 minutes
    Cooking Time: 30 minutes

SALSA

1 16-oz. can tomatoes, drained and chopped fine
1 7-oz. can diced green chilies
1/2 teaspoon minced garlic
1/4 teaspoon Tabasco sauce
1/2 teaspoon basil
1/2 onion, chopped
1 tablespoon wine vinegar
1 teaspoon parsley flakes
1/2 teaspoon Mrs. Dash
1/2 teaspoon seasoned pepper

Combine all ingredients, stirring well. Can be used as a dip, relish, or baked
potato topping. If you use a blender, use 2 of the tomatoes; blend well with
onion and green pepper. Add remaining ingredients and mix slightly. Tasty
with homemade or fat-free commercial corn chips.
    Servings: variable
    Preparation Time: 15 minutes
    Cooking Time: none

CHIP DIP-PIZZA SAUCE

2 cups diced onions
1 tablespoon minced garlic
1 28 oz. can tomato sauce
1 tablespoon basil
1/2 teaspoon oregano
1/2 teaspoon salt
1/4 teaspoon pepper
1/8 teaspoon Tabasco sauce
1/8 teaspoon fennel seed
1/4 teaspoon thyme leaves

Combine all ingredients in saucepan and simmer for 45 to 60 minutes.
Refrigerate or freeze for future use.

MEXICAN HOT SAUCE OR DIP

1 29-oz. can tomato puree
3/8 teaspoon oregano
3/8 teaspoon Tabasco sauce
4 1/2 teaspoon lemon juice
3/8 teaspoon black pepper
1 1/2 teaspoon chili powder
3/4 teaspoon garlic powder
3/8 teaspoon cumin
3/8 teaspoon salt
3/8 teaspoon red pepper
1 teaspoon red wine vinegar

Combine all ingredients. Keeps well in the refrigerator for up to 2 weeks and freezes well. Makes a wonderful chip dip.
     Servings: variable
     Preparation Time: 15 minutes
     Cooking Time: none

RICE MILK

4 cups water
1 cup cooked brown rice

In a blender container place 1 cup of cooked brown rice, add 4 cups water, blend until smooth and milky. Refrigerate in a quart jar. Shake before using. (You can now buy Fat-Free Rice Milk, it's good).
NOTE: For milk only let set for 1 hour then pour off milk and use sediment in stews, soups and gravy. You may want to add 1 teaspoon vanilla per quart for better taste.
     Servings: makes 1 quart
     Preparation Time: 5 minutes

Hundreds of Common Foods...

Percent of Fat—Protein—Carbohydrate and Cholesterol Milligram Content

Few people know the caloric percentage content (fat, protein, and carbohydrate) or the amount of cholesterol contained in the foods they eat. To help you be a wise consumer, values for many foods are shown on the following table. Percentages are not always equal to 100 percent because of the baseline data used. Calculations used: 1 gram fat = 9 calories, 1 gram protein and carbohydrate = 4 calories. These are rounded figures creating over or under 100%. U.S. Department of Agriculture figures in grams are also rounded. In spite of these rough figures you can quickly determine which foods provide low fat (10 percent or less), protein (10-15 percent), and about (80 percent) complex carbohydrate. All data was obtained from the U.S. Department of Agriculture publication, Home and Garden Bulletin Number 72, Nutritive Value of Foods, 1988.

Caloric Percentages
tr = trace

Food	% Fat	% Protein	% Carbo- hydrate
Artichokes	2%	22%	87%
Asparagus, cuts and tips	2%	44%	71%
Avocado	88%	5%	15%
Almonds	79%	14%	14%
Apricots	2%	8%	96%
Apples, unpeeled without cores	tr	tr	100%
Apples, with cores	7%	tr	100%
Banana	3%	3%	100%
Bacon (3 med. slices 16 mg. chol.)	74%	22%	tr
Barley, raw	3%	9%	90%

Food	% Fat	% Protein	% Carbo-hydrate
Beef			
chuck, roasted (3 oz. 87 mg. chol.)	72%	27%	0%
ground, broiled (3 oz. 76 mg. chol.)	66%	32%	0%
sirloin, broiled (3 oz. 77 mg. chol.)	56%	38%	0%
rib, roasted (3 oz. 72 mg. chol.)	74%	24%	0%
Beans, Pinto	3%	23%	74%
Beans, Great Northern	4%	27%	72%
Beans, Lima	3%	25%	75%
Beets, sliced	tr	15%	80%
Black-eyed peas	4%	27%	74%
Blackberries, raw	5%	5%	96%
Blueberries, raw	5%	5%	100%
Brazil nuts, shelled	92%	8%	8%
Bread, whole wheat 100%	13%	17%	74%
Bread, oatmeal	16%	13%	74%
Broccoli	6%	44%	80%
Brussels Sprouts	8%	40%	80%
Bulgur , uncooked	4%	13%	86%
Butter (1/2 cup, 247 mg. chol.)	100%	0.4%	tr
Cashew nuts	74%	10%	22%
Cabbage	tr	26%	80%
Cabbage, Chinese	tr	40%	80%
Carrots	tr	13%	93%
Cauliflower	tr	32%	80%
Celery	tr	20%	80%
Cheese:			
Natural:			
Blue (1 oz. 21 mg. chol.)	72%	24%	4%
Camembert (1 1/3 oz. 27 mg. chol.)	70%	27%	tr
Cheddar (1 oz. 30 mg. chol.)	73%	24%	1%
Cottage:			
Creamed, (4%)(1 cup 34 mg. chol.)	38%	48%	10%
Low-fat, (2%) (1 cup 19 mg. chol.)	18%	60%	15%

Food	% Fat	% Protein	% Carbohydrate
Uncreamed, dry curd, less than (1/2% fat) (1 cup 10 mg. chol.)	7%	80%	9%
Cream cheese (1 oz. 31 mg. chol.)	90%	8%	4%
Feta (1 oz. 25 mg. chol.)	72%	21%	5%
Mozzarella, made with:			
whole milk (1 oz. 22 mg. chol.)	67%	30%	5%
part skim milk (1 oz. 15 mg. chol.)	56%	40%	5%
Muenster (1 oz. 27 mg. chol.)	77%	26%	tr
Parmesan, grated (1 tbsp. 4 mg. chol.)	72%	32%	tr
Provolone (1 oz. 20 mg. chol.)	72%	28%	4%
Ricotta, made with:			
whole milk (1 cup 124 mg. chol.)	67%	26%	6%
part skim milk (1 cup 76 mg. chol.)	50%	33%	15%
Swiss (1 oz. 26 mg. chol.)	69%	30%	3%
Pasteurized Process Cheese:			
American (1 oz. 27 mg. chol.)	77%	23%	tr
Swiss (1 oz. 24 mg. chol.)	66%	29%	4%
Food, American (1 oz. 18 mg. chol.)	72%	25%	8%
Spread, American (1 oz. 16 mg. chol.)	74%	25%	10%
Cream, sweet:			
Half and half (1 cup 89 mg. chol.)	80%	8%	12%
Light, coffee (1 cup 159 mg chol.)	90%	tr	8%
Whipping, light (1 cup 265 mg chol.)	95%	2%	4 %
Whipping, heavy (1 cup 326 mg chol.)	96%	4%	tr
Sour (1 cup 102 mg chol.)	87%	5%	8%

Note: One cup of half and half contains 17.3 grams (62 percent) saturated fat. One cup of whipping cream contains 54.8 grams (62 percent) saturated fat. One cup of sour cream contains 30 grams (62 percent) saturated fat. One cup of pressurized whipped topping contains 8.3 grams of saturated fat. Saturated fat causes destruction of the blood vessels and the body makes additional cholesterol from saturated fat.

Food	% Fat	% Protein	% Carbohydrate
Cherries	8%	8%	88%
Chestnuts	8%	6%	86%
Chickpeas	13%	22%	66%

Food	% Fat	% Protein	% Carbo-hydrate
Chicken:			
breast, no skin, roasted			
(3 oz. 73 mg. chol.)	19%	77%	0%
breast, batter dipped, fried			
(4.9 oz. 119 mg. chol.)	44%	38%	14%
drumstick, roasted			
(1.6 oz 41 mg. chol.)	24%	64%	0%
drumstick, fried			
(2.5 oz. 62 mg. chol.)	51%	32%	12%
Chocolate, baking or bitter	83%	8%	22%
Chocolate candy, milk, plain	56%	5%	44%
Chocolate candy, milk, peanuts	64%	15%	35%
Clams, raw meat (3 oz. 43 mg. chol.)	14%	67%	12%
Coconut meat	85%	3%	17%
Collards, frozen	15%	33%	80%
Corn chips (commercial fried)	52%	5%	41%
Corn, frozen kernels	tr	14%	99%
Corn, sweet, ear	10%	14%	89%
Corn, canned whole kernel	5%	12%	89%
Crab meat, canned (1 cup 135 mg. chol.)	20%	68%	2%
Cranberry juice, sweetened	tr	tr	100%
Cucumbers	tr	tr	95%
Dates	tr	3%	100%
Eggs, raw:			
whole (1 egg 274 mg. chol.)	66%	30%	5%
white (0 mg. chol.)	tr	80%	tr
yolk (1 yolk 272 mg. chol.)	83%	18%	tr
Eggs, cooked:			
fried in butter (1 egg 278 mg. chol.)	66%	25%	4%
hard cooked, (1 egg 274 mg. chol.)	67%	30%	5%
poached (1 egg 273 mg. chol.)	67%	30%	5%
scrambled or omelet, with milk			
and butter (1 egg 282 mg. chol.)	65%	25%	7%
Eggplant, steamed	tr	16%	96%

Food	% Fat	% Protein	% Carbo-hydrate
Endive, raw	tr	40%	80%
Filberts (hazelnuts), chopped	89%	8%	10%
Figs (medium)	3%	5%	100%
Flounder, without added fat			
(3 oz. 59 mg. chol.)	11%	85%	tr
Flounder, with butter			
(3 oz. 68 mg. chol.)	45%	53%	tr
Flounder, with margarine			
(3 oz. 55 mg. chol.)	45%	53%	tr
Grapes	tr	tr	100%
Grapefruit	tr	4%	98%
Honey	0%	0%	100%
Kale, raw, chopped	20%	22%	70%
Kiwi fruit	tr	8%	97%
Lamb, lean and fat:			
chops, braised (2.2 oz 77 mg. chol.)	61%	36%	0%
loin, broiled (2.8 oz. 78 mg. chol.)	61%	37%	0%
leg, roasted (3 oz. 78 mg. chol.)	57%	43%	0%
rib, roasted (3 oz. 77 mg. chol.)	23%	74%	0%
Lemons	tr	16%	100%
Lentils	4%	29%	70%
Lettuce	13%	28%	62%
Liver, cooked (3 oz. 410 mg. chol.)	34%	50%	15%
Margarine, regular	100%	.04%	.04%
Mangos	7%	3%	100%
Milk and Milk Products:			
Whole milk (1 cup 33 mg. chol.)			
(Whole milk 64% saturated fat)	48%	21%	29%
Low-fat (2%) no milk solids added			
(Low Fat (2%) 58% saturated fat)			
(1 cup 18 mg. chol.)	38%	26%	40%
Low-fat (1 %) no milk solids added			
(low-fat (2%) 58%saturated fat)			
(1 cup 10 mg. chol.)	27%	32%	48%

Food	% Fat	% Protein	% Carbo-hydrate
Non-fat (skim) no milk solids added (1 cup 5 mg. chol.)	tr	38%	56%
Buttermilk (1 cup 9 mg. chol.) (Buttermilk 65% saturated fat)	18%	32%	48%
Canned:			
Whole (1 cup 74 mg. chol.) (Whole milk 62% saturated fat)	50%	20%	29%
Skim (1 cup 9 mg. chol.)	4%	38%	58%
Dried:			
Buttermilk	14%	35%	51%
Non-fat, instant (3.2 oz 17 mg. chol.)	3%	39%	58%
Milk Beverages:			
Cocoa and chocolate-flavored prepared (8 oz. whole milk plus 3/4 oz.powder 33 mg. chol.)	36%	16%	53%
Powder, non-fat dry (1 oz 1 mg. chol.)	9%	12%	88%
Eggnog, commercial (1 cup 149 mg. chol.)	50%	12%	39%
Malted milk (8 oz. whole milk plus 3/4 oz. powder 34 mg. chol.)	38%	14%	46%
Milk Desserts, Frozen:			
Ice cream, regular about (11% fat butterfat) (1 cup 59 mg. chol.)	48%	7%	47%
Soft serve frozen custard, rich about (16% butterfat) (1 cup 88 mg. chol.)	61%	5%	37%
Ice Milk, vanilla, about 4% butterfat (1 cup 18 mg. chol.)	28%	11%	63%
Yogurt:			
Low-fat, plain (8 oz. 14 mg. chol.)	25%	33%	44%
Non-fat (8 oz. 4 mg. chol.)	tr	41%	54%
Whole milk yogurt (8 oz. 29 mg. chol.)	45%	22%	31%

Food	% Fat	% Protein	% Carbo-hydrate

Caution, remember: One cup of whole milk contains 8 grams of fat, 64 percent of which is saturated. One cup of low-fat (2%) milk contains 5 grams of fat, 58 percent of which is saturated. Most all dairy beverages and frozen desserts average about 60 percent saturated fat, including low-fat products.

Food	% Fat	% Protein	% Carbohydrate
Melons, raw:			
Cantaloupe	9%	8%	92%
Honeydew	tr	8%	100%
Mushrooms, raw	tr	20%	60%
Mustard greens, cooked	tr	60%	60%
Nectarines, raw	14%	6%	98%
Oatmeal	12%	17%	69%
Okra	tr	32%	96%
Olives	99%	tr	tr
Onions, raw, chopped	tr	15%	87%
Onions, raw, spring	tr	40%	80%
Oranges	tr	7%	100%
Ocean perch, breaded, fried (3 oz. 66 mg. chol.)	54%	35%	15%
Oysters, raw (1 cup 120 mg. chol.)	23%	50%	20%
Papayas, raw	tr	6%	100%
Parsnips, cooked	tr	6%	96%
Peaches	tr	11%	100%
Peanuts, dry roasted	79%	12%	16%
Peanuts, roasted in oil	82%	11%	14%
Peanut butter	76%	21%	12%
Pears, raw with skin	9%	4%	100%
Peas, green, canned, drained	8%	28%	73%
Peas, green, frozen	tr	26%	75%
Peas, split, dry, cooked	4%	28%	73%
Pecans, halves	91%	4%	11%
Peppers, sweet, raw	tr	20%	80%
Peppers, hot, chili, raw	tr	20%	80%
Pineapple, raw	12%	5%	100%

Food	% Fat	% Protein	% Carbo- hydrate
Pine nuts, pinon, shelled	96%	8%	13%
Pistachio nuts, dry, shelled	76%	15%	17%
Plums	tr	tr	100%
Pork, fresh, cooked			
Chops, loin, broiled			
(3.1 oz. 84 mg. chol.)	62%	35%	0%
Chops, loin, pan fried			
(3.1 oz. 92 mg. chol.)	73%	25%	0%
Ham, leg, roasted (3 oz. 79 mg. chol.)	65%	34%	0%
Rib, roasted (3 oz. 69 mg. chol.)	67%	31%	0%
Potatoes, baked or broiled	tr	9%	93%
Potatoes, fried in oil	45%	5%	50%
Potatoes, au gratin	53%	15%	34%
Potatoes, scalloped	43%	9%	54%
Potato salad, with mayonnaise	53%	8%	31%
Potato chips	60%	4%	38%
Prunes, dried	tr	3%	100%
Pumpkin, canned	11%	19%	94%
Radishes	tr	tr	80%
Raspberries	15%	7%	93%
Rice, brown, cooked	4%	9%	87%
Rice, white	tr	7%	89%
Salmon:			
Canned, pink (3 oz. 34 mg. chol.)	38%	57%	0%
Baked, red (3 oz. 60 mg. chol.)	32%	60%	0%
Smoked (3 oz. 51 mg. chol.)	48%	48%	0%
Sardines (3 oz. 85 mg. chol.)	46%	46%	0%
Scallops, breaded, frozen			
(3 oz. 70 mg. chol.)	46%	32%	21%
Sesame seeds, dry, hulled	80%	18%	9%
Shrimp, french fried			
(3 oz. 168 mg. chol.)	45%	32%	22%
Soybeans, dry, cooked, drained	35%	34%	32%
Spaghetti, white, cooked	5%	15%	82%

Food	% Fat	% Protein	% Carbo-hydrate
Spinach, cooked	tr	50%	70%
Squash, cooked, summer	26%	23%	91%
Squash, baked, winter	11%	10%	90%
Strawberries, raw	9%	9%	89%
Sunflower seed, dry, hulled	79%	15%	13%
Sweet potatoes, baked	tr	7%	97%
Tangerines	tr	11%	100%
Tomatoes, raw	tr	16%	80%
Trout, broiled with butter and lemon juice (3 oz. 71 mg. chol.)	46%	48%	tr
Turkey, light and dark, roasted (3 oz. 45 mg. chol.)	35%	57%	12%
Tuna, canned solids, drained:			
Oil pack, chunk light (3 oz. 55 mg. chol.)	38%	58%	0%
Water pack, solid white (3 oz. 48 mg. chol.)	7%	89%	0%
Tuna salad (1 cup 80 mg. chol.)	46%	35%	20%
Turnips, cooked, diced	tr	13%	100%
Turnip greens, cooked, drained	tr	27%	80%
Veal, rib, roasted (3 oz. 109 mg. chol.)	55%	40%	0%
Walnuts, pieces or chips	86%	9%	11%
Watermelon	12%	8%	90%
Wheat flour, whole	5%	16%	85%
Wheat flour, white, enriched	2%	11%	83%
White flour, cake or pastry	3%	8%	89%
Yeast, bakers, dry, active	tr	60%	60%

Caloric Percentages and Cholesterol Content of Common Mixed Food Dishes

Food	% Fat	% Protein	% Carbo- hydrate	% Chol- esterol
Entrees				
Beef and vegetable stew, home recipe, 1 cup	45%	29%	27%	71 mg.
Beef pot pie, baked, 1/3 of 9" pie	52%	16%	30%	42 mg.
Chicken a la king, 1 cup	65%	23%	10%	221 mg.
Chicken and noodles, 1 cup	44%	24%	28%	103 mg.
Chicken chow mein, home recipe, 1 cup	35%	49%	16%	75 mg.
Chicken pot pie, home recipe, 1/3 of 9" pie	51%	17%	31%	56 mg.
Chili con carne with beans, canned, 1 cup	42%	22%	36%	28 mg.
Chop suey with beef or pork, home recipe, 1 cup	51%	35%	17%	68 mg.
Macaroni and cheese, home recipe, 1 cup	46%	16%	37%	44 mg.
Quiche Lorraine, 1 slice, 1/8 of 8" pie	72%	9%	19%	285 mg.
Spaghetti with meatballs, home recipe, 1 cup	33%	23%	47%	89 mg.
Soups				
Canned, condensed, prepared with equal volume of milk:				
Clam chowder, New England, 1 cup	38%	22%	41%	22 mg.
Cream of chicken, 1 cup	52%	15%	32%	27 mg.
Cream of mushroom, 1 cup	61%	12%	29%	20 mg.
Tomato, 1 cup	34%	15%	55%	22 mg.
Canned, condensed, prepared with equal volume of water:				
Bean with bacon, 1 cup	32%	28%	54%	3 mg.

Food	% Fat	% Protein	% Carbo-hydrate	% Chol-esterol
Grain Dishes				
French toast, 1 slice	15%	41%	44%	112 mg.
Muffins, 2 1/2 in. diam., 1 1/2" high				
Blueberry, 1 muffin	33%	9%	59%	19 mg.
Bran, 1 muffin	43%	10%	61%	24 mg.
Corn, 1 muffin	31%	8%	58%	23 mg.
Noodles, egg, 1 cup	9%	14%	74%	50 mg.
Noodles, chow mein, canned, 1 cup	45%	11%	47%	5 mg.
Pancakes, 4 in. diameter:				
Buckwheat, from mix with				
buckwheat and enriched flours,				
egg and milk added, 1 pancake	33%	15%	44%	20 mg.
Plain from mix, 1 pancake	30%	13%	53%	16 mg.
Waffles, made with enriched flour,				
7 in. diameter, 1 waffle	48%	11%	42%	102 mg.
Baked Desserts				
Cakes from mixes with enriched flour:				
Angel food, tube, 1/12 of cake	tr	10%	92%	0 mg.
Coffee cake, crumb, 7 3/4 in. x				
5 5/8 in. x 1 1/4 in. cake	27%	8%	66%	279 mg.
Devil's food with chocolate frosting:				
2 layer, 8 in. diameter, whole	27%	5%	68%	598 mg.
1 piece, 1/16 of cake	27%	5%	68%	37 mg.
Yellow with chocolate frosting:				
2 layer, 8 in. diameter, whole	30%	5%	68%	576 mg.
1 piece, 1/16 of cake	30%	5%	68%	36 mg.
Carrot, with cream cheese frosting,				
1 piece, 1/16 of cake	49%	4%	49%	74 mg.
Plain sheet cake without frosting:				
whole cake	34%	5%	61%	552 mg.
1 piece, 1/9 of cake	34%	5%	61%	61 mg.
Cheesecake, commercial:				
Whole cake, 9 in. diameter	57%	7%	37%	2053 mg.
1 piece, 1/12 of cake	57%	7%	37%	170 mg.

Food	% Fat	% Protein	% Carbo-hydrate	% Chol-esterol
Baked Desserts (cont.)				
Brownie with nuts, frosting, home recipe,				
1 3/4 in. x 1 3/4 in. x 7/8 in.	57%	5%	46%	18 mg.
Cookies made with enriched flour:				
Chocolate chip, home recipe,				
2 1/3 in. diam., 4 cookies	54%	4%	56%	18 mg.
Oatmeal with raisins,				
2 5/8 in. diam., 4 cookies	37%	5%	58%	2 mg.
Peanut butter, home recipe,				
2 5/8 in. diam., 4 cookies	51%	13%	45%	22 mg.
Sugar cookie from refrigerator				
dough, 2 1/2 in. diam., 4 cookies	46%	3%	52%	29 mg.
Danish pastry, packaged, made with				
white flour, plain, one 12 oz. ring	48%	6%	46%	292 mg.
Doughnuts, white flour:				
cake, plain, 3 1/4 in. diam., 1 in.				
high, 1 doughnut	51%	12%	45%	20 mg.
yeast, leavened, glazed, 3 3/4 in.				
diam., 1 1/4 in. high,				
1 doughnut	50%	12%	44%	21 mg.
Pie crust made with enriched flour,				
vegetable shortening, baked:				
Home recipe, 9 in. diam. shell	60%	5%	38%	0 mg.
Mix, 9 in. diam., 2 crust pie	56%	5%	38%	0 mg.
Pies:				
Apple, 1 pie	40%	3%	59%	0 mg.
Blueberry, 1 pie	40%	4%	58%	0 mg.
Cherry, 1 pie	40%	4%	59%	0 mg.
Creme, 1 pie	45%	3%	52%	46 mg.
Custard, 1 pie	46%	11%	44%	1010 mg.
1 piece, 1/6 of pie	46%	11%	44%	169 mg.
Lemon meringue, 1 pie	35%	6%	60%	817 mg.
1 piece, 1/6 of pie	35%	6%	60%	143 mg.
Pecan, 1 pie	50%	5%	49%	569 mg.
Pumpkin, 1 pie	48%	8%	46%	655 mg.
1 piece, 1/6 of pie	48%	8%	46%	95 mg.

Major Fast Foods:
Fat % and Grams,
Cholesterol—Sodium—Calorie Content

Note: This nutritional information was obtained from each Fast Food Company's latest published material. Fat percentages were calculated by multiplying fat grams times 9 (there are approximately 9 calories in every gram of fat), then dividing the total fat calories by the total calories of the item. The percentage of total fat is important to know, and hopefully will be on all food labeling soon.

FAST FOOD	Fat Grams	% of FAT	Choles. (mg.)	Sodium (mg.)	Total Calories
MCDONALD'S (1994 Statistics)					
Big Mac.	26	**45%**	75	930	510
Quarter Pounder w/cheese	29	**50%**	95	1160	520
Quarter Pounder	20	**43%**	70	690	420
McChicken Sandwich	29	**53%**	50	800	490
Filet-O-Fish	16	**42%**	35	710	360
McLean Delux w/cheese	16	**35%**	70	1040	400
Cheeseburger	13	**38%**	40	770	320
Chicken McNuggets (6)	18	**55%**	65	530	300
Chicken McNuggets (9)	27	**53%**	95	800	450
Chef Salad	11	**48%**	180	730	210
Ranch Salad Dressing (1 pkg)	21	**78%**	20	550	230
Sausage McMuffin w/egg	29	**59%**	255	820	440
Sausage Biscuit w/egg	35	**62%**	245	1200	520
Bacon, Egg & Cheese Biscuit	27	**56%**	240	1310	450
Biscuit	13	**46%**	0	840	260
Cheese Danish Muffin	22	**49%**	70	340	410

FAST FOOD	Fat Grams	% of FAT	Choles. (mg.)	Sodium (mg.)	Total Calories
BURGER KING (1994 Statistics)					
Whopper Sandwich	39	**56%**	90	850	630
Whopper w/cheese	46	**58%**	115	1270	720
Double Whopper	56	**58%**	170	920	860
Double Whopper w/cheese	63	**60%**	195	1340	950
Whopper Jr. w/cheese	28	**54%**	75	760	460
Hamburger	10	**35%**	30	500	260
Cheeseburger	14	**43%**	45	710	300
Double Cheese w/bacon	39	**55%**	145	1200	640
BK Big Fish Sandwich	43	**54%**	60	1090	720
Chicken Sandwich	43	**54%**	60	1400	700
Chicken Tenders (6)	12	**44%**	35	530	250
French Fries (med.)	20	**45%**	0	240	400
Onion Rings	14	**42%**	0	810	310
Dutch Apple Pie	15	**45%**	0	230	310
Croissan'wich w/sausage egg & cheese	41	**70%**	255	1000	530
Croissan'wich w/bacon egg & cheese	24	**63%**	225	790	350
French Toast Sticks	27	**48%**	0	496	500
Ranch Dressing	19	**94%**	10	170	180
Ranch Dipping Sauce	17	**94%**	0	200	170
WENDY'S (1994 Statistics)					
Single w/everything	23	**45%**	75	860	440
Big Bacon Classic	36	**52%**	110	1500	640
Jr. Bacon Cheeseburger	25	**52%**	65	870	440
Cheeseburger Kid's Meal	13	**39%**	45	770	310
Chicken Club Sandwich	25	**44%**	75	990	520
French Fries (med.) 4.6 oz	17	**44%**	0	210	340
Cheddar Cheese, shredded	6	**71%**	15	110	70
Chicken Nuggets	20	**64%**	50	600	280
Chocolate Chip Cookie	13	**43%**	15	260	280
Baked Potatoes Bacon & Cheese	18	**30%**	20	1280	530

FAST FOOD	Fat Grams	% of FAT	Choles. (mg.)	Sodium (mg.)	Total Calories
Cheese	23	36%	30	610	560
Sour Cream 1 pkt.	6	83%	10	15	60
Margarine 1 pkt.	5	83%	—	—	60
Plantarian:					
Plain Large Potato	0	0%	0	25	310
TACO BELL (1994 Statistics)					
Chicken Soft Taco	10	40%	58	553	223
Soft Taco	11	45%	32	539	223
Soft Taco Supreme	15	52%	47	551	268
Taco	11	56%	32	276	180
Taco Supreme	15	58%	47	287	225
Tostado	11	41%	14	593	242
7 Layer Burrito	21	39%	28	1115	485
Bean Burrito	12	28%	5	1138	391
Beef Burrito	19	39%	57	1303	432
Big Beef Burrito Supreme	25	42%	72	1418	525
Burrito Supreme	19	38%	47	1184	520
Chicken Burrito Supreme	23	38%	125	1130	520
Chili Cheese Burrito	18	41%	47	980	391
Nachos Bell Grande	34	47%	49	952	633
Nachos Supreme	27	66%	18	471	367
Mexican Pizza	38	59%	50	1003	574
Nachos	18	46%	9	398	345
Taco Salad	55	58%	79	1132	838
Light Soft Taco	5	28%	25	—	180
Light Bean Burrito	6	18%	5	—	330
Light 7 Layer Burrito	9	18%	5	—	440
PIZZA HUT (1 slice of medium pizza, 1994 Statistics)					
Cheese Pizza	8	37%	25	534	205
Beef Pizza	11	41%	26	709	229
Ham Pizza	7	32%	32	591	184

FAST FOOD	Fat Grams	% of FAT	Choles. (mg.)	Sodium (mg.)	Total Calories
Pepperoni Pizza	10	42%	25	627	215
Italian Sausage	12	46%	31	650	236
Pork Topping	12	44%	26	709	237
Meat Lover's	13	40%	39	892	288
Veggie Lover's	7	33%	17	545	186
Pepperoni Lover's	16	49%	42	862	289
Supreme	13	45%	31	795	257
Super Supreme	14	48%	35	880	270
Plantarian Pizza:	est.	est.		est.	est.
(No cheese or added fat, use olives sparingly, if any, 4 or 5 vegetable topping with sauce—tastes great, low in fat)	1	12%	0	350	90
SUBWAY (1994 Statistics)					
Spicy Italian Roll	63	54%	137	3020	1043
BMT Sub-Honey Wheat Roll	57	50%	133	3199	1011
Cold Cut Combo Sub-Italian Roll	41	42%	166	2278	883
Subway Club Salad	19	49%	84	1979	346
Tuna Sub-Italian Roll	72	59%	85	1498	1103
Tuna Salad	68	81%	85	760	756
Seafood & Crab-Hon. Wheat Roll	58	52%	56	2027	1015
Seafood & Crab Salad	53	73%	66	1229	639
Meatball Sub-Honey Wheat Roll	45	43%	88	2082	947
Steak & Cheese Sub-Hon. Wht Roll	33	41%	82	1616	711
Turkey Breast Sub-Hon. Wht Roll	20	27%	67	2520	674
Turkey Breast Salad	16	48%	67	1732	297
Ham & Cheese Sub-Hon. Wht. Roll	22	30%	73	2508	673
Veg & Cheese Sub-Hon. Wht Roll	18	29%	19	1136	565
Plantarian	est.	est.	est.	est.	est.
Veggie—Sub-Honey Wheat Roll	3	10%	0	340	250

(No animal Food, No mayo, No olives, heavy on tomatoes; also peppers, lettuce, onions, other veggies, pickles, mustard.)

FAST FOOD	Fat Grams	% of FAT	Choles. (mg.)	Sodium (mg.)	Total Calories
KENTUCKY FRIED CHICKEN (1994 Statistics)					
Original Recipe					
Quarter Breast & Wing	19	**50%**	157	1104	335
Quarter Thigh & Leg	24	**64%**	163	980	333
Breast	20	**50%**	115	870	360
Thigh	17	**58%**	110	570	260
Wing	8	**53%**	40	380	150
Extra Crispy					
Breast	28	**53%**	80	930	470
Thigh	25	**59%**	70	540	370
Wing	13	**60%**	45	290	200
Chicken Sandwich	27	**50%**	47	1060	482
Kentucky Nuggets (6)	18	**57%**	66	865	284
Hot Wings (6)	33	**63%**	150	1230	471
Corn on the Cob	12	**47%**	0	76	222
Macaroni & Cheese	8	**46%**	16	531	162
Red Beans & Rice	3	**23%**	4	315	114
Buttermilk Biscuit	12	**52%**	2	564	200
Cornbread (1)	13	**51%**	42	194	228
Mashed Potatoes & Gravy	5	**41%**	1	386	109
Cole Slaw	6	**47%**	5	177	114
Garden Rice*	1	**11%**	0	576	75

*This is an acceptable item for a Plantarian however, it is high in salt.

FAST FOOD	Fat Grams	% of FAT	Choles. (mg.)	Sodium (mg.)	Total Calories
DAIRY QUEEN (1994 Statistics)					
Homestyle Hamburger	12	**38%**	45	630	290
Homestyle Cheeseburger	17	**44%**	55	850	340
Homestyle Double Cheeseburger	31	**52%**	115	1130	540
Homestyle Ultimate Burger	43	**58%**	135	1210	670
Cheese Dog	18	**55%**	40	950	290
Fish Fillet Sandwich w/Cheese	21	**45%**	60	850	420
Chicken Breast Sand. w/Cheese	25	**48%**	70	980	480
French Fries Regular	14	**40%**	0	160	300
Regular Vanilla Cone	10	**26%**	30	140	340

FAST FOOD	Fat Grams	% of FAT	Choles. (mg.)	Sodium (mg.)	Total Calories
Regular Vanilla Shake	16	24%	50	260	600
Hot Fudge Brownie Delight	29	37%	35	340	710
Reg. Heath Blizzard	36	40%	60	410	820
Regular Yogurt Cone	0	0%	5	115	260
Small Yogurt Straw. Sunday	0	0%	0	80	200
Small Strawberry Breeze	0	0%	5	115	290
Dairy Queen Yogurt is FAT FREE					
ARBY'S (1991 Statistics)					
Reg. Roast Beef	14.8	37%	39	588	353
Beef 'N Cheddar	19.9	39%	52	955	451
French Dip	12.2	31%	47	678	345
Roast Chicken Deluxe	19.5	47%	20	913	373
Turkey Deluxe	20.2	45%	39	1047	399
Ham 'N Cheese	14.7	40%	45	1350	330
Garden Salad	8.6	52%	74	99	149
Potato Cakes	12.8	53%	0	397	204
Jamocha Shake	10.5	25%	35	262	368

Further Reading 231

Further Reading

McDougall Books

"The McDougall Plan," by John A. McDougall, M.D. and Mary A. McDougall, New Century Publishers, 1983.

"McDougall's Medicine: A Challenging Second Opinion," by John A. McDougall, M.D., New Century Publishers, 1985.

"The McDougall Program: Twelve Days to Dynamic Health," by John A. McDougall, M.D., National Books Publisher, 1990.

"The McDougall Program for Maximum Weight Loss" by John McDougall, M.D., Plume Publishing, 1995, N.Y., N.Y.

"The McDougall Health-Supporting Cookbooks," Volume 1 and 2, by Mary McDougall, 1986.

Barnard Books

"The Power of Your Plate," by Neal D. Barnard, M.D., Book Publishing Company, Summertown, Tennessee, 1990. Write P.O. Box 6322, Washington, D.C. 20015.

"Food for Life," by Neal B. Barnard, M.D., Harmony Books, N.Y., N.Y., 1993.

"Foods that Cause You To Lose Weight"-"The Negative Calorie Effect," by Neal Barnard, 1994.

Ornish Books

"Dr. Dean Ornish's Program for Reversing Heart Disease," by Dean Ornish, M.D., Random House, 1990.

"Stress, Diet and Your Heart," by Dean Ornish, M.D., Signet Books, 1983.

"Eat More Weigh Less," by Dean Ornish M.D., Harper Collins Publisher Inc, N.Y., N.Y., 1993.

Whitaker Books

"Reversing Heart Disease," by Julian M. Whitaker, M.D., Warner Books Publisher, 1985.

"Reversing Diabetes," by Julian M. Whitaker, M.D., Warner Books Publisher, 1987.

"Reversing Health Risks," by Julian M. Whitaker, M.D., G. P. Putnam's Sons, New York, 1988.

"Dr. Whitakers Guide to Natural Healing," Julian Whitaker, M.D., Prime Press, Rockland, CA, 1994.

Pritikin Books

"The Pritikin Program for Diet and Exercise," by Nathan Pritikin with Patrick M. McGrady, Jr., Bantam Books Publisher, 1979.

"The Pritikin Promise: 28 Days to a Longer, Healthier Life," by Nathan Pritikin, Simon and Schuster, 1983.

"Diet for Runners," by Nathan Pritikin, New York: Simon and Schuster, 1985.

"Pritikin: The Man Who Healed America's Heart," by Tom Monte with Ilene Pritikin, Rondale Publishers, 1988.

"The New Pritikin Program," by Robert Pritikin, Simon and Schuster Publishers, 1990.

Robbins Books

"Diet for a New America," by John Robbins, Stillpoint Publishing, Walpole, N.H. 03608, 1987.

"May All Be Fed, Diet for a New World," by John Robbins, William Morrow Co., N.Y., N.Y., 1992.

Sorenson Book

"MegaHealth," by Dr. Marc Sorensen, Ed. D.
National Institute of Fitness, Publisher, 202 N. Snow Canyon Rd., Ivans, Ut. 84738, 1992.

Alabaster Book

"The Power of Prevention," by Oliver Alabaster, M.D., Saville Books, 1989, Washington, D.C., Georgetown 20007.

China Study

Cornell-China-Oxford Project on Nutrition, Health and Environment, Diet, Lifestyle and Mortality in China: A Study of the Characteristics of 65 Countries by J. Chen, T. Colin Campbell, J.L. and R. Petro. Published jointly by Oxford University Press, Cornell University Press, and The China People's Medical Publishing House, 1990. Contact Cornell University Press for ordering information at P.O. Box 6525, Ithaca, NY 14850.

Cooper Books

"Controlling Cholesterol," by Kenneth H. Cooper, M.D., Bantam Books Publisher, 1988.

"Aerobics," by Kenneth H. Cooper, M.D., Bantam Books Publisher, 1968.

Relaxation Control

"The Relaxation Response," by Herbert Benson, M.D., Avon Publishing, 1975.

"Beyond the Relaxation Response," by Herbert Benson, M.D. with William Proctor, Berkeley Publishing, 1984.

"Love Is Letting Go of Fear," by Gerald G. Jampolsky, M.D., Bantam Books, 1981.

"Inner Peace, Inner Power," by Dr. Nelson Boswell, Fawcett Gold Medal, Ballantine Books, 1985.

"What to Say When You Talk to Yourself," by Shad Helmstetter, Ph.D., Pocket Books, 1986.

"The Complete Guide to Your Emotions and Your Health," by Emrika Padus and the Editors of Prevention Magazine, Rodale Press, Emmanus, PA, 1986.

"Dr. Dean Ornish's Program for Reversing Heart Disease," by Dean Ornish, M.D., Random House, 1990.

"Stress, Diet and Your Heart," by Dean Ornish, M.D., Signet Books, 1983.

The NEW Four Food Groups 1991

Physicians Committee for Responsible Medicine, a National Organization, headquarters, 5100 Wisconsin Avenue N.W., Suite 404, Washington, D.C. 20016. Telephone: (202) 686-2210. Neal D. Barnard, M.D., President.

Misleading Labels

Time Magazine, July 15, 1991, The Fight Over Food Labels, pp. 52-55.

Eat Your Beans

Newsweek, May 20, 1991, Nutrition, pp. 70-71.

Magazine Articles

Time Magazine, January 14, 1991, Breast Cancer, A Puzzling Plague, pp. 48-52.

"A New Menu to Heal the Heart: A yearlong study proves that diet, exercise and stress reduction can open arteries and save lives," by Dr. Dean Ornish, Newsweek Magazine, July 30, 1990.

"Can Lifestyle Changes Reverse Coronary Heart Disease?" by Dr. Dean Ornish, et al, Lancet 336:129-133, July 21, 1990.

U.S. News and World Report, August 6, 1990, "Reversing Heart Disease," pp. 54-61.

Newsweek Magazine, December 10, 1990, "Politics of Breast Cancer," pp. 62-68.

Readers' Digest, "Good News About Your Heart," (Feb., 1991) p. 23-31.

Guide to Healthy Eating, Sept.-Oct. 1990, PROTEIN:Exploding the Myths, Physicians Committee for Responsible Medicine, P.O. Box 6322, Washington, D.C., 20016.

Guide to Healthy Eating, May-June 1991, Poultry: What You Don't Know Could Kill You, Physicians Committee for Responsible Medicine, Publishers.

Health and Healing, Phillips Publishing, Inc., 7811 Montrose Road, Potomac, MD 20854. Call 1-800-777-5005.

Facts and Figures

American Heart Association, 1995 Heart and Stroke Facts.

American Cancer Society, Cancer Facts and Figures, 1995.

Rate of Diabetes as Underlying Cause of Death.

Nutritive Value of Foods, Home and Garden Bulletin Number 72, United States Department of Agriculture.

Morbidity and Mortality Weekly Report, Centers For Disease Control, Dept. of Health and Human Services, Atlanta, GA.

Diabetes: Facts You Need To Know, American Diabetes Association, National Center, Alexandria, VA.

Miscellaneous

"Get the Fat Out," Victoria Moran, Crown Publishing, N.Y., N.Y., 1994.

"Take It Off Keep It Off, " Dr. Art Ulene, M.D., Ulysses Press, Berkely CA, 1995.

"The Word of Wisdom Food Plan," by Kenneth E. Johnson Sr., M.D., Publishers, S.L.C., UT, 1993.

"The 10% Solution-for a Healthy Life," by Raymond Kurzweil, Crown Publishing, Inc., N.Y., N.Y., 1993.

"Understanding And Managing Cholesterol," by Kevin P. Bryne, M.D., Human Kinetics Books Publisher, Champaign, IL., 1991.
"Dr. Siegal's Natural Fiber Permanent Weight-Loss Diet," by Sanford Siegal, M.D., The Dial Press Publishers, 1975.
"The Truth About Fiber in Your Food," by Lawrence Galton, Crown Publisher, Inc., 1976.
"The Saccharine Disease," by T. L. Cleave M.R.C.P., Keats Publishing Inc., 1974.

References

References: Introduction

[1] Burkitt, D., "Some Diseases Characteristic of Modern Western Civilization," BR MED J1:274, 1973.

[2] McDougall Video Tape 1990.

[3] Kevin P. Byrne, M.D., Understanding and Managing Cholesterol, A Guide for Wellness Professionals (Champaign, IL: Human Kinetic Books, 1991), 287-89; Denver Post, Front Page, Lead Story, April; 9, 1991, report released by the National Cholesterol Education Program, Dr. Claude Lenfant, director of The National Heart, Lung and Blood Institute, sponsor of the education program.

References: Chapter One
Easy Permanent Weight Loss

[1] Denver Post, Front Page, Lead Story, April 9, 1991; The Physicians Committee for Responsible Medicine, Dr, Neal Barnard, president of the Physicians Committee, Virginia Messina, nutritionist editor of the bi-monthly magazine "Guide To Healthy Eating", 5100 Wisconsin Ave., N.W. Suite 404, Washington, D.C., 20016, Phone: 202-686-2210.

[2] Neal D. Barnard, M.D., The Power of Your Plate (Summertown, TN:Book Publishing Company, 1990), Chapters 1, 2, 6; Kevin P. Byrne, M.D., Understanding and Managing Cholesterol, A Guide for Wellness Professionals (Champaign, IL: Human Kinetics Books, 1991).

[3] Dr. Marc Sorenson, "MegaHealth," National Institute of Fitness, Publishers, Chapter 1, 1991. Victoria Moran, "Get the Fat Out," Crown Publishers, N.Y., N.Y., 1994. Neal Barnard, M.D., "Food For Life," Harmony Books, N.Y., N.Y. 1993, Chapter 4, 1993.

[4] Neal Barnard, M.D., "Food For Life," Harmony Books, N.Y., N.Y. 1993, Chapter 4, pages 85–111. Dr. Marc Sorenson, "MegaHealth," National Institute of Fitness Publishers, 1992, pages 14–84.

[5] Neal Barnard, M.D., "Food For Life," 1993, pages 94–96.

[6] Neal Barnard, M.D., "Food For Life," 1993, page 98. Dr. Marc Sorenson, "MegaHealth," 1992, pages 19–40.

References: Chapter Two
"The Miracle Diet" Program

[1] Diabetes Forecast, December 1990, A Publication of the American Diabetes Association, Inc. "Who Gets Diabetes?: pages 40-41; EastWest, September 1990. Volume 20, Number 9, The Champion Diet, by Nathaniel Mead, page 3. Tufts University Diet Nutrition Letter, Volume 8, No. 7, September 1990, Special Report, page 3. Nutrition Action Health Letter, Lessons from China, by Bonnie Liebman, page 1, 5-7.

[2] Neal D. Barnard M.D., The Power of Your Plate (Summertown, TN:Book Publishing Company, 1990), 7-10, 25-28; New Four Food Groups, Whole Grains, Vegetables, Legumes, Fruits, April 8, 1991. Physicians Committee for Responsible Medicine, 5100 Wisconsin Ave., N.W. Suite 404, Washington D.C., Ph. 202-686-2210; Arizona Republic April 9, 1991, Front Page and page four, T. Colin Campbell, professor of nutritional biochemistry at Cornell University.

[3] John A. McDougall and Mary A. McDougall, The McDougall Plan (Piscataway, NJ:New Century Publishers, 1983), 95; Neal D. Barnard M.D., The Power of Your Plate (Summertown, TN:Book Publishing Company, 1990), 183.

[4] John A. McDougall, The McDougall Program, Twelve Days to Dynamic Health (New York:NAL Books, 1990), 383-384; John A. McDougall, McDougall's Medicine:A Challenging Second Opinion (Piscataway NJ:New Century Publishers, 1985), 72-77.

[5] Adapted from John A. McDougall and Mary A. McDougall, The McDougall Plan (Piscataway NJ:New Century Publishers, 1983), 95.

[6] Guide to Healthy Eating, September-October 1990, Protein: Exploding The Myths, pages 2-3; Neal D. Barnard M.D., "The Power of Your Plate" (Summertown, TN:Book Publishing Company, 1990), 61-62, 81-82, 128-133, 183.

[7] T.B. Osborn and L.B. Mendel, "Amino acids in nutrition and growth", Journal of Biological Chemistry 17 (1914):325ff; John A. McDougall and Mary A. McDougall, The McDougall Plan (Piscataway, NJ:New Century Publishers, 1983), 96-99.

[8] John A. McDougall and Mary A. McDougall, The McDougall Plan (Piscataway, NJ: New Century Publishers, 1983), 100-101. Determined by grams per milliliter not as percentage of calories.

[9] John A. McDougall and Mary A.McDougall, The McDougall Plan (Piscataway, NJ: New Century Publishers, 1983), 55, 105. Determined as percentage of calories; Neal D. Barnard M.D., The Power of Your Plate (Summertown, TN:Book Publishing Company, 1990), 128-132.

[10] William Rose, "The Amino Acid Requirements of Adult Man," Nutrition Abstracts and Reviews 27:631,1957. For a brief summary of some of Rose's studies see John A. McDougall and Mary A. McDougall, The McDougall Plan (Piscataway, NJ:New Century Publishers, 1983) 97-99.

[11] H. Trowell, "Definition of Dietary Fiber and Hypotheses That It Is a Protective Factor in Certain Diseases," Am J Clin Nutr 29:417, 1976; D.Burkitt, "Some Diseases Characteristic of Modern Western Civilization," Br Med J1:274, 1973: D. Burkitt, "Dietary Fiber and Disease," JAMA 229:1068,1974. Nathan Pritikin, The Pritikin Program for Diet and Exercise (New York: Bantam Books, 1979) 364-386; Neal D. Barnard M.D., The Power of Your Plate (Summertown, TN:Book Publishing Company, 1990), 7-10, 13-18, 51-55, 69, 73-96, 117-127, 128-139.

[12] Dr. T. Colin Campbell, The Cornell-China-Oxford Project on Nutrition, Health and Environment. Cornell University, Division of Nutritional Sciences, Ithaca, N.Y. 14853. Ph. 607-255-1033.

[13] Research News Science, Vol. 1 248, by Anne Simon Moffit, May 4, 1990.

[14] Saturday Evening Post, China's Blockbuster Diet Study, by Jane Brody Oct. 1990. pages 30-32.

[15] Nutritional Action Health Letter, Lessons from China by Bonnie Liebman, pages 1, 5-7, December 1990, Vol. 17, No. 10, Center for Science in the Public Interest.

[16] Science Times, The New York Times, May 8, 1990, Huge Study of Diet Indicts Fat and Meat, by Jane Brody.

[17] EastWest, Sept. 1990, The Champion Diet, by Nathaniel Mead, pages 44-50, 98, 99, 102, 104.

[18] Nathan Pritikin, The Pritikin Program for Diet and Exercise (New York:Bantam Books, 1979) 9, 11, 28, 35; Julian M. Whitaker, Reversing Heart Disease (New York:Warner Books, 1985) 73, 79; John A. McDougall and Mary A. McDougall, The McDougall Plan (Piscataway, NJ: New Century Publishers, 1983), 34, 63, 116-122: Newsweek, July 30, 1990, Page 59, last paragraph. American Health, The Worlds Healthiest Diet, by Susan S. Lang, September 1989, pages 105-107, 110, 112; Neal D. Barnard M.D.,

The Power of Your Plate (Summertown, TN: Book Publishing Company, 1990), 73-96.

[19] A sampling from the extensive listing in Appendix One in this book.

[20] Reprinted from Bulletin of The Walter Kempner Foundation (Durham, N.C.) Vol. 4, No. 1, June 1972. This weight chart shows what Dr. Kempner considers reasonable weight for people of different heights, who do not have diabetes mellitis, heart, kidney or blood vessel disease, or disturbances in fat metabolism, etc. Patients with such complications should, of course, have weights 10-15% lower.

References: Chapter Four
Herbivores versus Carnivores

[1] Funk and Wagnall's New Encyclopedia #5, p. 314.

[2-6] John A. McDougall, M.D., The McDougall Newsletter, Volume 5, No. 5, Sept/Oct 1991. John A. McDougall and Mary A. McDougall, The McDougall Plan (Piscataway, NJ: New Century Publishers, 1983), 27-28. Julllian M. Whitaker, M.D., *99 Secrets for a Longer Healthier Life* (Phillips Publishing Inc., 7811 Montrose Rd., Potomac, MD 20854), 2-4. Dr. Marc Sorenson, *MegaHealth,* National Institute of Fitness, Ivins, UT, 1992, Chapter 7, Herbivorous by Design, pgs. 311-331. John Robbins, *Diet for a New America* (Stillpoint Publishing, Box 640, Walpole, NH 03608), p. 258-260.

[7] Webster's Ninth New Collegiate Dictionary, "Primate: any of an order of mammals comprising man together with the apes and monkeys" p. 934. See also Funk and Wagnall's New Encyclopedia #21, "Primate: suborder Anthropoidea, comprising monkeys, apes, and humans," p. 274.

[8] Julian M. Whitaker, M.D., *99 Secrets for a Longer Healthier Life* (Phillips Publishing Inc., 7811 Montrose Rd, Potomoac, MD 20854), 2-4. See also John A. McDougal and Mary A. McDougall, The McDougall Plan (Piscataway, NJ: New Century Publishers, 1983), p. 37-38. John Robbins, *Diet for a New America,* (Stillpoint Publishing, 1987), pages 214–217.

[9] Dr. Marc Sorenson, *MegaHealth,* p. 316.

References: Chapter Five
Cholesterol Kills

[1] Kevin P. Bryne, M.D., Understanding And Managing Cholesterol (Champaign, IL: Human Kinetics Books, 1991), 288; John A. McDougall, McDougall's Medicine:A Challenging Second Opinion (Piscataway, NJ: New Century Publishers, 1985), 98-99.

[2] Heart and Stroke Facts (Dallas, TX:American Heart Association, 1994).

[3] John A. McDougall, M.D., McDougall's Medicine: A Challenging Second Opinion (Piscataway, NJ: New Century Publishers, 1985), 144-60; John A. McDougall, The McDougall Program, Twelve Days to Dynamic Health (New York: NAL Books, 1990), 352-55.

[4] John A. McDougall, McDougall's Medicine: A Challenging Second Opinion (Piscataway, NJ: New Century Publishers, 1985), 157; and Julian M. Whitaker, Reversing Heart Disease (New York: Warner Books, 1985, Hardcover edition), 78-84.

[5] John A. McDougall, M.D., The McDougall Tapes, Heart Disease Prevention and Cure, Tape 2, sides A, B. Neal D. Barnard M.D., The Power of Your Plate (Summertown, TN:Book Publishing Company, 1990), 14-15.

[6] Julian M. Whitaker, M.D., Reversing Heart Disease (New York: Warner Books, 1985, hardback edition), 96-97.

[7] John A. McDougall and Mary A. McDougall, The McDougall Plan (Piscataway, NJ: New Century Publishers, 1983), 63.

[8] Neal D. Barnard M.D., The Power of Your Plate (Summertown, TN:Book Publishing Company, 1990), 16-23; Kevin P. Bryne, Understanding And Managing Cholesterol (Champaign, IL: Human Kinetics Books, 1991), 6-9.

[9] John A. McDougall, Heart Disease Prevention, (Audio Tape 2, Side 1, 1989); John A. McDougall, McDougall's Medicine: A Challenging Second Opinion (Piscataway, NJ: New Century Publishers, 1985), pages 106-107.

[10] Dean Ornish et al., "Can lifestyle changes reverse coronary heart disease?" Lancet 336 (July 21, 1990): 129. See also Dean Ornish, Dr. Dean Ornish's Program for Reversing Heart Disease (New York: Random House, 1990).

[11] Dean Ornish, M.D., "A new menu to heal the heart: A yearlong study proves that diet, exercise and stress reduction can open arteries and save

lives," Newsweek (July 30, 1990): 58-59; and Joanne Silberner, "Reversing Heart Disease," U.S. News & World Report (August 6, 1990): 54-61.

[12] Dr. Allan Brett, Harvard Medical School, is quoted in Dean Ornish's book, "Dr. Dean Ornish's Program for Reversing Heart Disease" (New York: Random House, 1990), 59. "Elevated cholesterol levels are very important in the genesis of atherosclerosis. Many genetic factors and environmental risk factors can increase or decrease the tolerance to elevated cholesterol levels." Ibid., 60.

[13] Neal D. Barnard M.D., The Power of Your Plate (Summertown, TN:Book Publishing Company, 1990), 24-28; D. Blankenhorn and D. M. Kramsch, "Reversal of atherosis and sclerosis," Circulation 79 (1989): 1. David Blankenhorn, "Prevention or reversal of atherosclerosis: Review of current evidence," American Journal of Cardiology 63 (1989): 38H.

[14] Julian M. Whitaker, Reversing Heart Disease (New York: Warner Books, 1985, hardback edition), 95-100, 105-6; John A. McDougall, McDougall's Medicine: A Challenging Second Opinion (Piscataway, NJ: New Century Publishers, 1985), 102-26; John A. McDougall and Mary A. McDougall, The McDougall Plan (Piscataway, NJ: New Century Publishers, 1983), 63-72; Robert Pritikin, The New Pritikin Program (New York: Simon and Schuster Publishers, 1990), 56-61, 70; Neal D. Barnard, M.D., The Power of Your Plate (Summertown, TN:Book Publishing Company, 1990), 13-30.

[15] John A. McDougall, Heart Disease Prevention, (Audio Tape 2, Side A, 1989). John A. McDougall, McDougall's Medicine: A Challenging Second Opinion (Piscataway, NJ: New Century Publishers, 1985), 98-99; Kevin P. Bryne, Understanding And Managing Cholesterol (Champaign, IL: Human Kinetics Books, 1991), 6, 288.

[16] John A. McDougall, McDougall's Medicine: A Challenging Second Opinion (Piscataway, NJ: New Century Publishers, 1985), 99, 142-143; Enos, W. "Pathogenisis of Coronary Disease in American Soldiers Killed in Korea" JAMA, 158:912, 1988.

[17] John A. McDougall, Heart Disease Prevention, (Audio Tape 2, Side 1, 1989); Neal D. Barnard M.D., The Power of Your Plate (Summertown, TN:Book Publishing Company, 1990), 16-17.

[18] Julian M. Whitaker, M.D., Reversing Heart Disease (New York: Warner Books, 1985), 10-11.

[19] Kevin P. Bryne, M.D., Understanding And Managing Cholesterol (Champaign, IL: Human Kinetics Books, 1991), 6-9.

[20] John A. McDougall, M.D., Heart Disease Prevention, (Audio Tape 2, Side 1, 1989); Julian M. Whitaker, Reversing Heart Disease (New York: Warner Books, 1985, paperback), 10-11, 80-83; Neal D. Barnard M.D., The Power of Your Plate (Summertown, TN:Book Publishing Company, 1990), 12-17.

[21] John A. McDougall, M.D., McDougall's Medicine: A Challenging Second Opinion (Piscataway, NJ: New Century Publishers, 1985), 125.

[22] Julian M. Whitaker, Reversing Heart Disease (New York: Warner Books, 1985), 11-12.

[23] Neal D. Barnard M.D., The Power of Your Plate (Summertown, TN:Book Publishing Company, 1990), 24; Julian M. Whitaker, Reversing Heart Disease (New York: Warner Books, 1985), 12.

[24] John A. McDougall, McDougall's Medicine: A Challenging Second Opinion (Piscataway, NJ: New Century Publishers, 1985), 119-21.

[25] Dr. Dean Ornish's Program for Reversing Heart Disease (New York: Random House, 1990); D. Blankenhorn, "Prevention or reversal of Atherosclerosis: Review of current evidence, " American Journal of Cardiology 63 (1989):38H; Neal D. Barnard M.D., The Power of Your Plate (Summertown, TN:Book Publishing Company, 1990), 24: Kevin P. Bryne, M.D., Understanding and Managing Cholesterol (Champaign, IL:Human Kinetics Books, 1991) 6-9.

[26] John Robbins, Diet For A New America, (Walpole, NH: Ph. 1-800-847-4014, Stillpoint Publishing, 1987), pages 308-325.

[27] Neal Barnard, M.D., "Food For Life" (Harmony Books, New York, New York, 1993) 50-51

John A. McDougall, M.D., "The McDougall Program for Maximum Weight Loss" (Plume Publishing, New York, New York, 1994) 150-156.

References: Chapter Six
Fats—The Dreaded Enemy

[1] Neal D. Barnard M.D., The Power of Your Plate (Summertown, TN:Book Publishing Company, 1990), 18, 22-28, 56-62, 74-79, 90, 95, 126,

162, 182.; Nathan Pritikin, The Pritikin Program for Diet and Exercise (New York: Bantam Books, 1979), 9, 11-16.

[2] John A. McDougall, M.D., and Mary A. McDougall, The McDougall Plan (Piscataway, NJ: New Century Publishers, 1983), 22-25.

[3] "The Miracle Diet", Appendix One, Calorie Ratios, Home and Garden Bulletin Number 72, Department of Agriculture, 1988. Neal D. Barnard M.D., The Power of Your Plate (Summertown, TN:Book Publishing Company, 1990), 18, 22-28, 56-62, 74-79, 90, 95, 126, 162, 182.

[4] Neal D. Barnard, M.D., The Power of Your Plate (Summertown, TN:Book Publishing Company, 1990), 74-96; John A. McDougall and Mary A. McDougall, The McDougall Plan (Piscataway, NJ: New Century Publishers, 1983), 21-25.

[5] John A. McDougall and Mary A. McDougall, The McDougall Plan (Piscataway, NJ: New Century Publishers, 1983),116-124; John Robbins, Diet For A New America (Walpole, NH: Stillpoint Publishing, 1987), 254-259, 284-287; Neal D. Barnard M.D., The Power of Your Plate (Summertown, TN:Book Publishing Company, 1990), 21-22, 59-61, 80, 117-125.

[6] Nathan Pritikin, The Pritikin Program for Diet and Exercise (New York: Bantam Books, 1979), 9, 11, 28, 35; John A. McDougall and Mary A. McDougall, The McDougall Plan (Piscataway, NJ: New Century Publishers, 1983), 34; Julian Whitaker, Reversing Heart Disease (New York: Warner Books, 1985, paperback), 73

[7] Dictionary definition on back cover, Miracle Diet

[8] John A. McDougall and Mary A. McDougall, The McDougall Plan (Piscataway, NJ: New Century Publishers, 1983), 77, 79, 81, 83-84; Neal D. Barnard M.D., The Power of Your Plate (Summertown, TN:Book Publishing Company, 1990), 18, 22-28, 56-62, 74-79, 90, 95, 126, 162, 182.

[9] John A. McDougall and Mary A. McDougall, The McDougall Plan (Piscataway, NJ: New Century Publishers, 1983), 85; Julian Whitaker, Reversing Diabetes (New York: Warner Books, 1987, paperback), 31, 38-41; Neal D. Barnard M.D., The Power of Your Plate (Summertown, TN:Book Publishing Company, 1990), 125-128.

[10] Julian Whitaker, Reversing Heart Disease (New York: Warner Books, 1985, paperback), 86-87; John A. McDougall, McDougall's Medicine: A Challenging Second Opinion (Piscataway, NJ: New Century Publishers,

1985), 123-125; John A. McDougall and Mary A. McDougall, The McDougall Plan (Piscataway, NJ: New Century Publishers, 1983), 77-80.

[11] Adapted from Julian M. Whitaker, M.D., Reversing Heart Disease (New York: Warner Books, 1985, paperback), 87-88.

[12] Nathan Pritikin, The Pritikin Program for Diet and Exercise (New York: Bantam Books, 1979), 11. Julian M. Whitaker, Reversing Heart Disease (New York: Warner Books, 1985, paperback), 88-91.

References: Chapter Seven
Milk: DOES It Do A Body Good?

[1] Nathaniel Mead, Natural Health, July/August 1994.

[2] Michael F. Jacobson in FDA's Regulations of Animal Drug Residues in Milk (Washington, DC: U.S. Government Printing Office, 1990), 3, italics added; see also 8. Michael F. Jacobson in FDA's Regulations of Animal Drug Residues in Milk (Washington, DC: U.S. Government Printing Office, 1990), 5; see also 9-10. Michael F. Jacobson in FDA's Regulations of Animal Drug Residues in Milk (Washington, DC: U.S. Government Printing Office, 1990), 9. Michael F. Jacobson in FDA's Regulations of Animal Drug Residues in Milk (Washington, DC: U.S. Government Printing Office, 1990), 9. Michael F. Jacobson in FDA's Regulations of Animal Drug Residues in Milk (Washington, DC: U.S. Government Printing Office, 1990), 9.

[3] Michael F. Jacobson in FDA's Regulations of Animal Drug Residues in Milk (Washington, DC: U.S. Government Printing Office, 1990), 12-13.

[4] "How Safe Is The Milk We Drink?" Washington Post, 1990.

[5] "The incidence of food allergy is much higher than most realize. Allergic disease. . .affects 25 percent of the population with about half of the allergens being food. . . . In the United States, food allergy concerns a population of 30 million individuals. In addition, intolerance to lactose is estimated to involve another 33 million." James C. Breneman, Basics of Food Allergy, 2d ed. (Springfield, IL: Charles C. Thomas, 1984), 12. Breneman continues, "95 percent of food allergies are unknown. They are masked as headache, nervous stomach, sinusitis, fainting spells, obesity, bedwetting, learning disabilities, gallstones, colitis, and numerous other diagnoses in those unfortunates who do not know of their food intolerance. In spite of numerous dairy advertisements that milk is the perfect food for everybody,. . . milk is the most prevalent food allergen." Ibid., 13. "Cows milk is the undis-

puted 'king' of the food allergens. It is not only the most common in all age groups, but also causes an unusually large variety of symptoms. . . The physician who watches constantly for milk allergy will find that it is amazingly common." Frederic Speer, Food Allergy, 2d ed. (Boston: John Wright, 1983), 121.

[6] E.J. Eastham and W.A. Walker, "Adverse effects of milk formula ingestion on the gastrointestinal tract—An update, "Gastroenterology 76 (1979): 365-74. I. Jakobsson and T. Lindberg, "Cow's Milk as a Cause of Infantile Colic in Breast-Fed Infants," Lancet 2 (1978): 437-39; T.M. Bayless et el., "Lactose and Milk Intolerance: Clinical Implications," New England Journal of Medicine 292 (1975): 1156-59. "It is no longer justifiable to assume that, as the dairy-industry advertising jingle stated, 'everybody needs milk.' Ibid., 1159.

[7]"Background Information on Lactose and Milk Intolerance," Nutrition Reviews 30 (1972): 175-76. T.Gilat, "Lactose Deficiency: The World Pattern Today," Israel Journal of Medical Sciences 15 (1979): 369-73; John A. McDougall, The McDougall Program, Twelve Days To Dynamic Health, (New York, NY:NAL Books, 1990), 37,48; John A. McDougall and Mary A. McDougall, The McDougall Plan (Piscataway, NJ:New Century Publishers, 1983), 49-52.

[8] Neal Barnard, "The Power of Your Plate" Summertown, TN: Book Publishing Company, 1990.

[9]John A. McDougall and Mary A. McDougall, The McDougall Plan (Piscataway, NJ:New Century Publishers, 1983), 52-53. Dr. McDougall gives many scientific references; here are three: A.R.P. Walker, "The human requirement for calcium: Should low intakes be supplemented?" American Journal of Clinical Nutrition 25 (1972): 518-30. "There is no unequivocal evidence that an habitually low intake of calcium is deleterious to man, or that an increase in calcium intake would result in clinically detectable benefits." Ibid., 526. "Symposium on human calcium requirements," Journal of the American Medical Association 185 (1963):588-93. H. Spencer et el., "Influence of dietary calcium intake on Ca47 Absorption in man," American Journal of Medicine 46 (1969): 197-205.

[10] E.M.E. Poskitt et al., "Diet, sunlight, and 25-hydroxy vitamin D in healthy children and adults," British Medical Journal 1 (1979): 221-23; T. Stamp et al., "Comparison of oral 25-hydroxycholecalciferol, vitamin D and ultraviolet light as determinants of circulating 25-hydroxyvitamin D," Lancet 1 (1977): 1341-43.

References: Chapter Eight
Osteoporosis: Our Love Affair with Meat, Eggs and Milk

[1] Harrison, *Principles of Internal Medicine*, 8th ed., vol. II, p. 2029.

[2] Licata, A., "Acute Effects of Dietary Protein on Calcium Metabolism in Patients with Osteoporosis," *J. Gerontol*, 36:14-19, (1982); Allen, Ll, "Protein Induced Hypercalciuria: A Long-term Study," *Am. J. Nutr.*, 32:741-749, (1979); Schuette, S., "Studies on the Mechanism of Protein-induced Hypercalciuria in Older Men and Women," *J. Nutr.*, 110:305-315, (1980): Hegsted, M., "Long-term Effects of Protein Intake on Calcium Metabolism in Young Adult Women," *J. Nutr.*, 111:224-251, (1981).

[3] Koop, C., *The Surgeon General's Report on Nutrition and Health*, United States Department of Health and Human Services, (Rocklin, CA: Prima Publishing and Communications, 1988); Orwall, E., "The Rate of Bone-Mineral Loss in Normal Men and the Effects of Calcium and Cholecalciferol Supplementation," *Ann. Intern. Med.*, 112:29-34, (1990); Ris, B., "Does Calcium Supplementation Prevent Postmenopausal Bone Loss," New Eng. J. Med., 316:173-177, (1987).

[4] Harrison, "Principle of Internal Medicine," 8th ed., vol.II, p. 2028.

[5] Rose, W., "The Amino Acid Requirements of Adult Man," *Nutrition Abstracts and Review*, 27:631; McLaren, D. "The Great Protein Fiasco," *Lancet*, 2:93, (1974); Irwin, M., "A Conspectur of Research on Protein Requirements of Man." *J. Nutr.*, 101:385, (1971); Abdulla, M., "Nutrient Intake and Health Status of Begans," *Am. J. Cin. Nutr.*, 34:2464, (1981).

References: Chapter Nine
Cancer Prevention—the Best Cure

[1] Cancer Facts and Figures—1995, (Atlanta, GA: American Cancer Society, 1995), 3; Brochure: The Great American Food Fight Against Cancer, "These three top cancer fighters can help you and your family reduce cancer risks—Fork, Knife, Spoon." American Cancer Society Inc., 1990. United States Dept. of Health and Human Services, The Surgeon General's Report on Nutrition and Health (Rocklin, CA: Prima Publishing and Communications, 1988), 178-79.

[2]John A. McDougall and Mary A. McDougall, The McDougall Plan (Piscataway, NJ:New Century Publishers, 1983), 183; John A. McDougall M.D., The McDougall Tapes, Tape 4, Side B, Cancer Treatment, 1989; Neal D. Barnard, M.D., The Power of Your Plate (Summertown, TN:Book Publishing Company, 1990), 51-53.

[3] John A. McDougall and Mary A. McDougall, The McDougall Plan (Piscataway, NJ:New Century Publishers, 1983), 184; John A. McDougall M.D., The McDougall Tapes, Tape 4, Side A-B, Cancer Prevention, Cancer Treatment 1989.

[4] American Cancer Society

[5] John A. McDougall M.D., The McDougall Tapes, Tape 4, Side A, Cancer Prevention, 1989; Neal D. Barnard, M.D., The Power of Your Plate (Summertown, TN:Book Publishing Company, 1990), 66-67.

[6] The Arizona Republic, Vegetables may help avert some cancers, page A1, A11, July 21, 1990.

[7] John A. McDougall M.D., The McDougall Tapes, Tape 4, Side A, Cancer Prevention, 1989.

[8] Neal D. Barnard, M.D., The Power of Your Plate (Summertown, TN:Book Publishing Company, 1990), 59-61; Burkitt, D.P. & Trowell, H.C. (1975). Refined carbohydrate foods and disease, New York; Academic Press; Trowell, H.C. (1978). The development of the concept of dietary fiber in human nutrition. American Journal of Clinical Nutrition, 31, S 3-S 11.

[9] Burkitt, D. (1984). Fiber as protective against gastrointestinal diseases. American Journal of Gastroenterology, 97, 249-252.

[10] Reddy, B., "Nutrition and Its Relationship to Cancer," Advances Cancer Research, 12:237-245, (1980).

[11] Burkitt, D., "Colon-Rectal Cancer: Fiber and Other Dietary Factors," Am. J. Clin. Nutr. 31:558-564, (1978); Freeman, H., "Dietary Fibre and Colonic Neoplasia," Can. Med. Assoc. 121:291-296, (1979).

[12] John A. McDougall M.D., The McDougall Tapes, Tape 4, Side A, Cancer Prevention, 1989.

[13] Newsweek, December 10, 1990, page 62.

[14] Time, January 14, 1991, page 49.

[15] John A. McDougall M.D., The McDougall Tapes, Tape 4, Side A, Cancer Prevention, 1989; Health Magazine, March 1991, Meals That Heal, pages 70-75; Kevin P. Bryne M.D., Understanding And Managing Cholesterol, A Guide for Wellness Professionals (Champaign, IL:Human

Kinetics Books, 1991), 184, 188-93; Neal D. Barnard, M.D., The Power of Your Plate (Summertown, TN:Book Publishing Company, 1990), 66-67.

[16] The Albuquerque Tribune, December 13, 1990, Red meat linked to colon cancer.

[17] Prevention and Nutrition, Feb. 1993.

[18] John A. McDougall M.D., The McDougall Tapes, Tape 4, Side A, Cancer Prevention, 1989; John A. McDougall and Mary A. McDougall, The McDougall Plan (Piscataway, NJ:New Century Publishers, 1983), 80, 82-84.

[19] Time, January 14, 1991, page 50.

[20] John A. McDougall M.D., The McDougall Tapes, Tape 4, Side A, Cancer Prevention, 1989.

[21] Armstrong, B., "Environmental Factors and Cancer Incidence and Mortality in Different Countries, with Special Reference to DietaryPractices," Int. J. Cancer, 15:617-631, (1975).

[22] Snowden, D., "Diet, Obesity, and the Risk of Fatal Prostate Cancer," Am. J. Epidemiol., 120:244-250, (1984); Hill, P., "Environmental Factors and Breast and Prostatic Cancer," Cancer Research, 41:3817-3818, (1981); Hill, P., "Plasma Hormones and Lipids in Men at Different Risk for Coronary Heart Disease," Am. J. Nutr., 33:1010-1018, (1980).

[23] Mills, P., "Cohort Study of Diet, Lifestyle, and Prostate Cancer in Adventist Men," Cancer 64:598-604, (1989). Neal Barnard, M.D., "Food For Life," Harmony Books, New York, New York, 50–51, 1993. Armstrong B, Doll R. "Environmental Factors and Cancer Incidence and Mortality in Different Countries, with Special Reference to Dietary Practices." Int J Cancer 1975; 15:617–31. Howell MA. "Factor Analysis of International Cancer Mortality Data and Per Capita Food Consumption." Br J Cancer 1974; 29:328–36. Rotkin ID. "Studies in the Epidemiology of Prostatic Cancer: Expanded Sampling." Cancer Treat Rep 1977; 61:173–80. Mettlin C., Selenskas S., Natarajan N., Huben R. "Beta-Carotene and Animal Fats and Their Relationship to Prostate Cancer Risk: A Case-Control Study. Cancer 1989; 64:605–12.

[24] Nathan Pritikin, The Pritikin Program for Diet and Exercise (New York: Bantam Books, 1979), 15; Robert Pritikin, The New Pritikin Program (New York: Pocket Books, 1991), 31-32; John A. McDougall M.D., The McDougall Tapes, Tape 4, Side A, Cancer Prevention, 1989.

[25] Nathan Pritikin, The Pritikin Program for Diet and Exercise (New York: Bantam Books, 1979), 18.

[26] John A. McDougall, McDougall's Medicine: A Challenging Second Opinion (Piscataway, NJ: New Century Publishers, 1985), 20-23; John A. McDougall and Mary A. McDougall, The McDougall Plan (Piscataway, NJ:New Century Publishers, 1983), 86-87; John A. McDougall M.D., The McDougall Tapes, Tape 4, Side A, Cancer Prevention, 1989.

[27] John A. McDougall M.D., The McDougall Tapes, Tape 4, Side A, Cancer Prevention, 1989.

[28] John Robbins, Diet For A New America (Walpole NH:Stillpoint Publishing 1987, 248-273; Saturday Evening Post, October, 1990, Diets That Protect Against Cancers In China, Pages 26-27; EastWest, September 1990, Volume 20, Number 9, The Champion Diet, Pages 44-50, 98-99, 102, 104; A scientific monograph on the Cornell-Oxford-China Project on Nutrition, Health and Environment. Contact Cornell University Press for ordering information at P.O. Box 6525, Ithaca, NY 14850:Phone; (607) 277-2211.

[29] Oliver Alabaster, M.D., The Power of Prevention (Saville Books, GeorgeTown, Washington, D.C., 1988) pages 13–15. Neal D. Barnard, M.D., The Power of Your Plate (Summertown, TN:Book Publishing Company, 1990), 68-72.

[30] Announced April 8, 1991, THE NEW FOUR FOOD GROUPS: The Physicians Committee For Responsible Medicine, 5100 Wisconsin Ave., N.W., Suite 404, Washington, D.C. 20016, (202) 686-2210, Neal D. Barnard, M.D., president.

[31] John A. McDougall M.D., The McDougall Tapes, Tape 4, Side A, Cancer Prevention, 1989

References: Chapter Ten
Diabetes and Diet

[1] American Diabetes Association, Diabetes: Facts And Figures, 1995.

[2] United States Dept. of Health and Human Services, The Surgeon General's Report on Nutrition and Health (Public Health Service Publication No. 88-50210), 4, 253-254; American Diabetes Association Management Letter, November 30, 1990; American Diabetes Association, Diabetes: Facts You Need To Know, 1990.

[3] Julian M. Whitaker M.D., Reversing Diabetes (New York: Warner

Books, 1987), 8-10, 31-41; John A. McDougall M.D., McDougall's Medicine: A Challenging Second Opinion (Piscataway, NJ: New Century Publishers, 1985), 210-214; Neal D. Barnard M.D., The Power of Your Plate (Summertown, TN:Book Publishing Company, 1990), 119-120, 125-128

[4] Prevention & Nutrition Magazine, July, 1992. Karjalainen J, Martin J.M., Knip, M; et al A bovine albumin peptide as a possible trigger of insulin-dependent diabetes mellitus, N Engl J. Med 1992:327:302-7. Scott, F.W. Cow milk and insulin-dependent diabetes mellitus: is there a relationship? Am. J. Clin-Nutr 1990:51:489-91

[5] Narva, A., "Research data on End Stage Renal Disease (ESRD) Among American Indians," *Indian Health Service Kidney Disease Program*, Albuquerque, NM (1990).

[6] Ringrose, H., "Nutrient Intakes in an Urbanized Micronesioan Population with a High Diabetes Prevalence," *Am. J. Clin. Nutr.*, 32:1334-1341, (1979).

[7] Ibid McDougall's Medicine 212-214; Julian M. Whitaker, Reversing Diabetes (New York: Warner Books, 1987), 31-41.

[8] United States Dept. of Health and Human Services, The Surgeon General's Report on Nutrition and Health (Public Health Service Publication No. 88-50210), 257-258: John A. McDougall, McDougall's Medicine: A Challenging Second Opinion (Piscataway, NJ: New Century Publishers, 1985), 214-215; Julian M. Whitaker, Reversing Diabetes(New York: Warner Books, 1987), 38-45.

[9] Ibid U.S. Surgeon General's Report, 259-260; Ibid McDougall's Medicine, 215-216. Julian M. Whitaker, Reversing Diabetes (New York: Warner Books, 1987), 42-45; Kevin P. Bryne M.D., Understanding And Managing Cholesterol, A Guide for Wellness Professionals (Champaign, IL:Human Kinetics Books, 1991), 187.

[10] United States Dept. of Health and Human Services, The Surgeon General's Report on Nutrition and Health (Public Health Service Publication No. 88-50210), 255-256; Julian M. Whitaker, Reversing Diabetes (New York: Warner Books, 1987), 9; Kevin P. Bryne M.D., Understanding And Managing Cholesterol, A Guide for Wellness Professionals (Champaign, IL:Human Kinetics Books, 1991), 154.

[11] John A. McDougall M.D., The McDougall Tapes, Tape 3, Side B, Blood Sludging, Diabetes, Hypoglycemia. John A. McDougall and Mary A.

McDougall, The McDougall Plan (Piscataway, NJ:New Century Publishers, 1983), 85.

[12] John A. McDougall M.D., The McDougall Tapes, Tape 3, Side B. Julian M. Whitaker, Reversing Diabetes (New York: Warner Books, 1987), 40-41; United States Dept. of Health and Human Services, The Surgeon General's Report on Nutrition and Health (Public Health Service Publication No. 88-50210), 263.

References: Chapter Eleven
High Blood Pressure—An Epidemic in America

[1] United States Dept. of health and Human Services, The Surgeon General's Report on Nutrition and Health (Rocklin, CA: Prima Publishing and Communications, 1988) 142.

[2] John A. McDougall, McDougall's Medicine: A Challenging Second Opinion (Piscataway, NJ: New Century Publishers, 1985), 177, 187-188; John A. McDougall and Mary A. McDougall, The McDougall Plan (Piscataway, NJ:New Century Publishers, 1983), 149-150; Julian M. Whitaker, Reversing Heart Disease (New York: Warner Books, 1985, paperback), 100-104.

[3] John A. McDougall M.D., The McDougall Tapes, Tape 3, Side A, Risk Factors: Obesity and High Blood Pressure.

[4] Ibid; John A. McDougall, McDougall's Medicine: A Challenging Second Opinion (Piscataway, NJ: New Century Publishers, 1985), 190 .

[5] Guide to Healthy Eating, Sept.-Oct. 1990, Salt:Should we shake the habit? page 6. Physicians Committee for Responsible Medicine; Julian M. Whitaker, Reversing Heart Disease (New York: Warner Books, 1985, paperback), 100-101; Kevin P. Bryne M.D., Understanding And Managing Cholesterol, A Guide for Wellness Professionals (Champaign, IL:Human Kinetics Books, 1991), 106.

[6] Nathan Pritikin, The Pritikin Program for Diet and Exercise (New York:Bantam Books, 1979), 46.

[7] John A. McDougall M.D., The McDougall Tapes, Tape 3, Side A, Risk Factors: Obesity and High Blood Pressure.

Kempner, W., "Treatment of Hypertensive Vascular Disease with Rice Diet," AMJ MED 4 (1948):545.

Kaplan, N., "Non-Drug Treatment of Hypertension: Review," ANN IN-TERN MED 102:359,1985.

[8]Julian M. Whitaker, Reversing Heart Disease (New York: Warner Books, 1985, paperback), 105-108; Kevin P. Bryne M.D., Understanding And Managing Cholesterol, A Guide for Wellness Professionals (Champaign, IL:Human Kinetics Books, 1991), 113-115. John A. McDougall, The McDougall Program, Twelve Days To Dynamic Health, (New York, NY:NAL Books, 1990), 363-366.

References: Chapter Twelve
Antioxidants—Nature's Cancer Killers—
Fight Free Radicals

[1] Dr. Julian M. Whitaker, M.D., Health & Healing
[2]Partners The News Magazine, Mar. 1995.

References: Chapter Thirteen
Millions Starve So We Can Eat Meat

[1] John Robbins, Diet For A New America (Walpole NH:Stillpoint Publishing 1987, ph. 1-800-847-4014), 350-51.

[2] Ibid: page 351.

[3]John Robbins, Diet For A New America (Walpole NH:Stillpoint Publishing 1987, ph. 1-800-847-4014), 352.

[4] Ibid: page 352.

[5] Ibid: page 353.

[6] John Robbins, Diet For A New America (Walpole NH:Stillpoint Publishing 1987, ph. 1-800-847-4014), 353-54; Denver Post, April 9, 1991, Page 1, Physicians Committee for Responsible Medicine Report, Washington, D.C.

[7] John Robbins, Diet For A New America (Walpole NH:Stillpoint Publishing 1987, ph. 1-800-847-4014), 357-59.

[8] Ibid: page 363.

[9] Ibid: page 367.

[10] John Robbins, Diet For A New America (Walpole NH:Stillpoint Publishing 1987, ph. 1-800-847-4014), 371-73.

[11] Arizona Republic, April 9, 1991, Front Page A1, A4; Denver Post, April 9, 1991, Page 1A, 8A.

[12] Denver Post, April 9, 1991, Page 1A, 8A; Arizona Republic, April 9, 1991, Page A1, A4.

[13] Guide to Healthy Eating, May-June 1991, pages 3-6, Physicians Committee for Responsible Medicine. Fisher, Irving, "The Influence of Flesh Eating on Endurance", Yale Medical Journal, 13 (5):205-221, 1907.

[14] Ioteyko, J., et al, Enquete Scientifique sur les vegetarians de Bruxelles, Henri Lamertin, Brussells, pg. 50.

[15] Astrand, Per-Olaf, Nutrition Today 3:No. 2, 9-11, 1968.

[16] Phillips, R. L., "Role of Life-style and Dietary Habits in Risk of Cancer Among Seventh-Day Adventists," Cancer Research, 1975; 35:3513-3522. See also Millo, P. et al, "Cohort Study of Diet, Lifestyle, and Prostate Cancer in Adventist Men," Cancer 1989, 64:605-612.

[17] Snowden, D., et al, *Diet, Obesity and Risk of Fatal Prostate Cancer*, American Journal of Epidemiology 1984, 120 (2);244-250. See also *Prostate Cancer A Preventable Disease*, Physicians Committee for Responsible Medicine Update News, Spring of 1992, Vol. 8, No. 1.

[18] David Snowden and R. L. Phillips, Phillips, *Does a Vegetarian Diet Reduce the Occurrence of Diabetes?* Am J Public Health, 1985; 75:507-517.

[19] *Castelli Speaks from the Heart*, AARP Bulletin, May 1992, Vol. 33 No. 5, p. 16.

[20] *Doctrine and Covenants* Section 89:10-16 (1833)

[21] Ezra Taft Benson, "In His Steps," Ensign Magazine (Sept. 1988).

For more information on The **"New Four Food Groups"** contact "The Physicians Committee for Responsible Medicine", 5100 Wisconsin Ave. N.W. Suite 404, (P.O. Box 6322) Washington, D.C. 20016. Phone: (202) 686-2210. Dr. Neal Barnard is president of the Physicians Committee.

References: Chapter Fourteen
Change: Making It All Work
With Diet and Exercise

[1] Nathan Pritikin, The Pritikin Program for Diet and Exercise (New York: Bantam Books, 1979), 35.

[2] Nathan Pritikin, Ibid: 14

[3] John McDougall, M.D., McDougall Program For Maximum Weight Loss (Plume, Penguin Books, N.Y., N.Y., 1995), 44–45.

[4] Kenneth H. Cooper, M.D., Aerobics (New York, NY: Bantam Books, 1968), 87–97; Lenore R. Zohman, M.D., Exercise Your Way To Fitness And Heart Health (Pamphlet, Best Foods, 1974).

[5] Dean Ornish, M.D., Dr. Dean Ornish's Program for Reversing Heart Disease (New York, NY: Random House, 1990).

[6] Herbert Benson, M.D., The Relaxation Response (New York, NY: Avon Books, 1975) 158–166.

[7] Emrika Padus and the Editors of Prevention Magazine, Your Emotions and Your Health (Emmaus, Penn: Rodale Press, Inc., 1986) 249–267.

References: Chapter Sixteen
Wise Consumers Know Their Numbers

[1] See Appendix One: Hundreds of Common Foods . . . % of Fat—Protein—Carbohydrate and Cholesterol Milligram Content. (*"The Miracle Diet."*)

[2] T. Colin Campbell et al, Diet, Lifestyle and Mortality in China, (publisher Cornell University Press) 1990, page 63.

General Index

Recipe Index

V

W

Z

You may indulge yourself and have a feast day
occasionally such as: Thanksgiving, Christmas, birthdays
and a few other celebrations but be sure to get right back
on the Plantarian Program so that you can
enjoy the
"Best Possible Health"
always.

Earl Updike

ABOUT THE AUTHOR

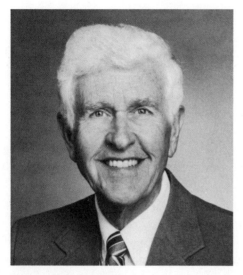

Earl F. Updike

Author Earl F. Updike is a businessman, writer, and a student of nutrition for over 50 years. He believes that the healthier you are, the better you can serve others.

He has taught for many years that everyone should follow a plant-centered food plan if you want to be thin and attractive. He also says that happiness and health are synonymous.

For half a century medical science has been proving by irrefutable evidence that the correct fuel for humans is plant food, just as it is for all primates.

Updike says, "If you want the 'Best Possible Health' you must eat a (starch) plant-based diet."

"The time has come to recognize that a plant-centered diet is the way of the future. 'The Miracle Diet' deals with the causes of degenerative diseases and reveals positive answers to weight loss and health. Read this book if you want the best possible health for yourself and your family."

Jack Anderson
Syndicated Columnist

"The three major killer diseases that now account for premature mortality are cancer, heart disease and stroke. They account for four out of five deaths in America. Yet these three diseases are *largely untreatable* and almost entirely preventable if we make right decisions.

Read this book and use the recipes. Practice prevention. Eating a plant-centered diet is the foundation of human health."

Oliver Alabaster, M.D.
Director, Institute of Disease Control
George Washington University Medical School

"This 'Plantarian' food plan has saved my life. After two heart by-pass surgeries I adopted 'The Miracle Diet' wholeheartedly. I now hike on mountain trails every morning and enjoy life.

Earl Updike's book reveals the secret of how to change from an animal laden, disease producing lifestyle to a 'new you.' By following the principles found in this book you will enjoy being lean and healthy for a lifetime."

Kenneth E. Johnson Sr., M.D.
Diplomate American Board of Internal Medicine

" 'The Miracle Diet' is nothing less than a prescription for a long disease-free life. Earl Updike shows us how a miracle takes place in our bodies when we adopt a Plantarian (plant-based) eating style. If you want to look and feel younger, lose weight and enjoy boundless health, read this book."

Dr. Marc Sorenson
Author— "MegaHealth"
National Institute of Fitness